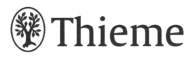

Functional and Selective Neck Dissection

Second Edition

Javier Gavilán, MD
Professor and Chairman
Department of Otorhinolaryngology
La Paz University Hospital
Madrid, Spain

Alejandro Castro, MD
Chief of Head and Neck Surgery Division
Department of Otorhinolaryngology
La Paz University Hospital
Madrid, Spain

Laura Rodrigáñez, MD
Head and Neck Surgeon
Department of Otorhinolaryngology
La Paz University Hospital
Madrid, Spain

Jesús Herranz, MD
Chief of Section
Department of Otorhinolaryngology
Complejo Hospitalario Universitario A Coruña
A Coruña, Spain

136 illustrations

Thieme
Stuttgart • New York • Delhi • Rio de Janeiro

Library of Congress Cataloging-in-Publication Data

Names: Gavilán, Javier, author. | Castro, Alejandro (Chief of Head and Neck Surgery Division), author. | Rodrigáñez, Laura, author. | Herranz, Jesús, author.

Title: Functional and selective neck dissection / Javier Gavilán, Alejandro Castro, Laura Rodrigáñez, Jesús Herranz.

Description: Second edition. | New York : Thieme, [2020] | Preceded by Functional and selective neck dissection / Javier Gavilán ... [et al.]. 2002. | Includes bibliographical references and index. | Summary: "This updated second edition presents a unique point of view based on fascial dissection techniques developed by several generations of renowned surgeons at La Paz University Hospital, Spain. This book lays a foundation with in-depth discussion of fascial compartmentalization of the neck. The text covers the evolution of modern neck dissection, from George Crile in 1906 to current cutting-edge procedures, and details the transition from radical neck dissection to a less aggressive, equally effective approach for treating lymph node metastases in head and neck cancer. The relationship between functional and selective neck dissection is discussed from a pragmatic and nonconventional perspective, elucidating the connection from historical, anatomic, and surgical standpoints. The four authors differentiate conceptual approaches, keystones in the evolution of scientific knowledge from surgical techniques, technical variations of a standard procedure designed to most effectively resolve a problem. The primary goal of this book is providing the reader with expert guidance on a full spectrum of fundamental surgical techniques"– Provided by publisher.

Identifiers: LCCN 2019054892 (print) | LCCN 2019054893 (ebook) | ISBN 9783132419537 (hardback) | ISBN 9783132419544 (ebook)

Subjects: MESH: Neck Dissection–methods | Head and Neck Neoplasms–surgery | Otorhinolaryngologic Surgical Procedures–methods Classification: LCC RD763 (print) | LCC RD763 (ebook) | NLM WE 708 | DDC 617.5/3–dc23

LC record available at https://lccn.loc.gov/2019054892

LC ebook record available at https://lccn.loc.gov/2019054893

Copyright © 2020 by Thieme Medical Publishers, Inc.

Thieme Publishers New York
333 Seventh Avenue, New York, NY 10001 USA
+1 800 782 3488, customerservice@thieme.com

Thieme Publishers Stuttgart
Rüdigerstrasse 14, 70469 Stuttgart, Germany
+49 [0]711 8931 421, customerservice@thieme.de

Thieme Publishers Delhi
A-12, Second Floor, Sector-2, Noida-201301
Uttar Pradesh, India
+91 120 45 566 00, customerservice@thieme.in

Thieme Revinter Publicações Ltda.
Rua do Matoso, 170 – Tijuca
Rio de Janeiro RJ 20270-135 - Brasil
+55 21 2563-9702
www.thiemerevinter.com.br

Cover design: Thieme Publishing Group
Typesetting by Thomson Digital, India

Printed in Germany by CPI Books GmbH   5 4 3 2 1

ISBN 978-3-13241-953-7

Also available as an e-book:
eISBN 978-3-13241-954-4

Important note: Medicine is an ever-changing science undergoing continual development. Research and clinical experience are continually expanding our knowledge, in particular our knowledge of proper treatment and drug therapy. Insofar as this book mentions any dosage or application, readers may rest assured that the authors, editors, and publishers have made every effort to ensure that such references are in accordance with **the state of knowledge at the time of production of the book.**

Nevertheless, this does not involve, imply, or express any guarantee or responsibility on the part of the publishers in respect to any dosage instructions and forms of applications stated in the book. **Every user is requested to examine carefully** the manufacturers' leaflets accompanying each drug and to check, if necessary in consultation with a physician or specialist, whether the dosage schedules mentioned therein or the contraindications stated by the manufacturers differ from the statements made in the present book. Such examination is particularly important with drugs that are either rarely used or have been newly released on the market. Every dosage schedule or every form of application used is entirely at the user's own risk and responsibility. The authors and publishers request every user to report to the publishers any discrepancies or inaccuracies noticed. If errors in this work are found after publication, errata will be posted at www.thieme.com on the product description page.

Some of the product names, patents, and registered designs referred to in this book are in fact registered trademarks or proprietary names even though specific reference to this fact is not always made in the text. Therefore, the appearance of a name without designation as proprietary is not to be construed as a representation by the publisher that it is in the public domain.

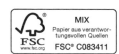

A Tribute to Osvaldo Suárez and César Gavilán

The following are the words of César Gavilán in the previous edition of this book:

The memory of Osvaldo Suárez, along with our gratitude, is still alive in the minds of those of us who had the privilege to meet him. We still remember his amazing surgical expertise, based on years of anatomical dissections. On the last day of his visit to Madrid he started a last case shortly before leaving for the airport. As the time of his plane's departure approached we offered to continue the case on our own. He gently declined saying that he could finish the case if he could operate without explaining the surgical details. We accepted his offer to see the scalpel in his hands literally fly over the surgical field in a way we had never seen before. The operation was completed in 20 minutes: 20 minutes of the cleanest, most effective surgery that we had ever seen.

He was not only a superb surgeon but also a great person with his colleagues and, especially, with his patients. His idea of function preservation always went hand in hand with a clear demarcation of priorities. His motto, "A life without voice is much better than a voice without life," stresses the importance of defining priorities in the field of laryngeal cancer treatment. We would like this book to be a tribute to his memory, often forgotten in the world of neck dissection.

César Gavilán passed away suddenly in 2004. We dedicate this second edition to his memory. Functional neck dissection is here because he was humble, visionary and dynamic. He accepted to see the surgery performed by one of the attendants to his course in Córdoba (Argentina) and immediately realized that the operation could be a major improvement for patients with laryngeal cancer. One year later Osvaldo Suárez spent two weeks in Madrid and functional neck dissection began to spread among European otorhinolaryngologists. He was also a great surgeon and teacher. His dedication to show the concept and surgical technique of functional neck dissection constitute the basis of the knowledge included in this book. Osvaldo Suárez and César Gavilán: two great men, two excellent surgeons. The origin of a new approach to neck dissection.

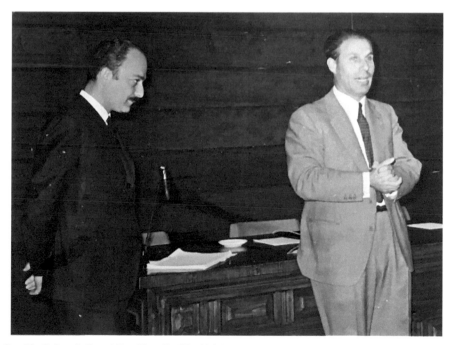

Dr. Osvaldo Suárez (left) and Dr. César Gavilán (right) at La Paz University Hospital in Madrid, Spain: 1969.

Contents

Foreword

The adverse prognostic impact of cervical lymph node metastases in head and neck cancer was appreciated by several pioneering surgeons in the first half of the 19th century. To address this problem, many attempts were made by Maximillian Von Chelius, J. C. Warren, Richard Von Volkmann, Theodor Kocher, and other noted persons to excise these metastatic lymph nodes; all unsuccessfully. At the turn of the 19th century, Sir Henry Trentham Butlin, in his Hunterian lecture, emphasized the need to excise upper cervical lymph nodes in the surgical treatment of tongue cancer. Franciszek Jawdynski from Poland has been credited with publishing the first report on neck dissection, in the Polish gazetta. However, the credit for reporting a systematic technique of excision of cervical lymph nodes from all levels in the neck for treatment of cancers of the head and neck goes to George Crile Sr., who published in the *Journal of the American Medical Association* in 1906 details of the operation of "radical neck dissection" based on his personal experience of 132 operations. Hayes Martin later popularized the operation and established it as the standard of surgical care for cervical lymph-node metastasis, and it remained in vogue for nearly three quarters of the 20th century. Although the operation was oncologically effective and considered the gold standard, it also caused significant esthetic and functional morbidity.

The authors of the second edition of this book bring a perspective from the experience of several generations of Latin surgeons largely influenced by the pioneering work of Oswaldo Suárez from Argentina and subsequent adoption of Suárez's system by César Gavilán in Spain and Ettore Boca in Italy, for the surgical management of cervical lymph nodes in head and neck cancer. The philosophy, goals, and principles of functional neck dissection and the technical details of respecting fascial planes form the backbone of the entire concept of functional and selective neck dissections. As the authors point out, selective neck dissections are a logical sequel to the concept of functional neck dissection, based on the knowledge of patterns of neck metastases. The concept of cervical lymphatics contained within the fascial compartments of the neck, initially developed and applied to surgical techniques by Dr. Suárez, is appropriately credited in this work. Subsequent promulgation of his concepts and techniques in Europe by César Gavilán and Ettore Bocca led to the accumulation of significant surgical experience, particularly in cancers of the larynx, to justify the validity of the concept and its surgical application with convincing outcomes. The authors propose functional neck dissection as a concept and not a modification of the standard radical neck dissection. To that end, the historical perspective detailed in this textbook is impressive.

Understanding of the patterns of cervical lymph-node metastasis has further advanced the concept of functional neck dissection to the development and clinical applicability of selective neck dissections. Thus, the varieties of selective neck dissections currently in vogue are called extensions of the concept, and a logical extension of the concept of functional neck dissection, as proposed in this book.

The authors are to be commended for putting together a fine contribution to the literature in the field of head and neck surgery and oncology. This book is a classic tour through the history of surgical management of neck metastasis and is a meticulous and outstanding treatise on the anatomy of the fascial planes in the neck, the cervical lymphatics, well illustrated with beautiful anatomic drawings by Laura Rodrigáñez and the technical aspects of the operation, its complications and their management. The years of experience amassed by the authors is reflected in the chapter on "Hints and Pitfalls." The addition of a chapter on frequently asked questions and answers is a refreshing nuance, which gives the impression of an interactive dialogue between the reader and the authors.

This opus from the surgical dynasty of the Gaviláns, now with support from Jesús Herranz and enhanced by contributions from Alejandro Castro and Dr. Rodrigáñez, representing the new generation of head and neck surgeons in Spain, is truly a monumental work on the history, development, philosophy, practice, and outcomes of functional neck dissection.

Jatin P. Shah, MD, PhD, DSc, FACS, FRCS(Hon), FRCSDS(Hon),
FDSRCS(Hon), FRCSI(Hon), FRACS(Hon)
E W Strong Chair in Head and Neck Oncology
Professor of Surgery
Memorial Sloan Kettering Cancer Center
New York, New York

Preface

The present book represents the philosophy and surgical technique of neck dissection used by the authors. It is based on the experience of several generations at La Paz University Hospital in Madrid, Spain, where functional neck dissection was introduced in Spain and in Europe in the late 1960s. It also describes the evolution of neck dissection during the 20th century, from George Crile to the surgery of the new millennium. Last but not least, it relates the transition from radical neck dissection to other less aggressive, but equally effective, procedures, which have been designed to manage the neck in patients with head and neck cancer.

The relation between functional neck dissection and selective neck dissection is approached from a pragmatic nonconventional perspective, which does not always follow the guidelines of the classifications currently used in the literature. However, by no means should this book be regarded as a proposal for a new classification of neck dissection. In fact, there is not even a chapter dedicated to the issue of neck dissection classification. Our main purpose is to clarify the connection between functional and selective neck dissection from historical, anatomic, and surgical standpoints. However, rest assured that this book is not limited to the history and philosophy of neck dissection; surgical technique constitutes a fundamental part of this volume. Surgical details are extensively demonstrated with sequential operative photographs of actual operations performed by the authors. Where necessary, line drawings are used to complement the details of the surgical field. The number of illustrations reflects the detail of the description provided.

A separate chapter on "hints and pitfalls" has been designed to provide the reader with technical guides and warnings that reflect the personal experience of the authors acquired through decades of practice. They are shared here to avoid repetition of previous mistakes. Many years ago, when I was in training, I learned from the late Antonio de la Cruz, MD, that to make science move forward you must be original in your own errors—this is the reason for this chapter.

Over the last 30 years we have been lecturing on neck dissection around the world. This has provided us with rich input from a variety of audiences concerning the most frequent doubts, problems, and demands regarding the various surgical techniques that are currently available. A separate chapter has been designed to answer the most frequently asked questions and to thereby make available to the reader a somehow more direct communication with the authors.

The conceptual approach to functional and selective neck dissection, the surgical indications for these procedures, and the operative technique demonstrated in this book express the ideas and opinions of the authors—a very small group of persons. Thus, the book should be regarded as a single-author work rather than as a multiauthored volume. Whereas there are many advocates for multiauthored books—as proven by their widespread diffusion in recent years—the clarity and uniform methodology of a surgical concept does not develop in a multiauthored book. To that extent, there is an obvious advantage in following the approach developed by one individual—or a small uniform group of experts—with years of authority in the field.

This book is primarily addressed to practicing head and neck surgeons involved in the management of malignant tumors. However, surgeons training in otorhinolaryngology, general surgery, or plastic surgery will also find it an interesting and valuable source of information. The graphic information included in the book will serve as a highly useful tool to familiarize readers with the procedure.

A major change can be found in the authors of this second edition of the book. César Gavilán, MD, my father, teacher, and faithful fellow for many years is no longer among us. My good old friend Lawrence W. DeSanto, MD, is retired and stays away from the field of science. Their place has been taken by the new ENT generation at La Paz University Hospital.

I emphasize that this book was written with the intention to clarify concepts and approximate postures in the controversial and sometimes contentious field of neck dissection. As often happens with conciliatory postures, the final result may be worse than the original situation. However, we assume the risk with the hope that the synthesizing approach to neck dissection that is given in this book may shed some light upon the field.

Prof. Javier Gavilán, MD
Professor and Chairman
Department of Otorhinolaryngology
La Paz University Hospital
Madrid, Spain

Acknowledgments

I acknowledge the efforts and dedication of the coauthors of this book. My thanks go first to my friend and "scientific brother" Jesús Herranz, MD. Over the years we have shared many hours of courses, discussions, and thoughts, which have culminated in this book. His energetic working capacity and critical compliance have been indispensable in the completion of this work. But the reason why this second edition is now in the shelves is the interest, dedication and hard work of the new coauthors. Alejandro Castro, MD, is like a son to me. He was my student at medical school, my resident on his early years, part of my staff later on, and right now he is the Chief of the Head and Neck Surgery Division at the Department of Otorhinolaryngology at La Paz University Hospital. I cannot think of a better person to whom to pass the torch of functional neck dissection.

I acknowledge the role of Laura Rodrigáñez, MD, on this second edition. She is one of these angels that seldom cross your way. I was lucky to be able to keep her in my team and right now she is the future of our head and neck surgery. She is not only a good surgeon but also a great illustrator. The best sample is within this book.

I would also like to express my sincere appreciation to those who have helped with this book. To all members of the Department of Otorhinolaryngology, fellows, residents, and nursing staff for their support and assistance with the clinical and surgical work associated with this book.

Last but not least, my thanks go to those who remain at home when I go to work and those who remain at the hospital when I come back home. My family and my patients are the two vital forces of my life. To my family for their love and support over the years, and to my patients who constitute the target of my efforts. Trying to cure them and improve their quality of life will remain as the unreachable utopia that I will always seek.

Prof. Javier Gavilán, MD
Professor and Chairman
Department of Otorhinolaryngology
La Paz University Hospital
Madrid, Spain

Introduction to the Second Edition

Functional and Selective Neck Dissection: the first thing a title like this would bring to my mind would be something like, "What is this book about?"; "What will I get from it?"; "Is this worth the try (money)?" More than 30 years ago we started to share our experience with functional neck dissection in head and neck cancer patients. At first, we were criticized for not being radical enough. Functional neck dissection was less than the standard cancer operation described by Crile; thus, its oncological safety was disputed. The years went by and we gradually witnessed a global shift toward less aggressive operations for early N stages. It seemed that the time for functional neck dissection had come. However, there was still criticism—now we were being too aggressive. It was time for selective neck dissections.

Throughout this period—when functional neck dissection was less than needed and when it apparently became more than required—we suspected that the problem was merely due to a lack of understanding of the concept of functional neck dissection. The operation is neither less aggressive than radical neck dissection nor more aggressive than selective neck dissection. It is simply different from radical neck dissection, and the basis for all types of selective neck dissections. Proving this is one of the main goals of this book.

There has been so much written about neck dissection in recent years that one can hardly believe there is still something new and interesting to add to the field. Thus, before we proceed, let us explain what we intend to present in this book, that is, what you can expect to find and what you will not find here.

What This Book Is About

Neck dissection has been evolving since 1906 when George Crile described the so-called radical neck dissection. From the very beginning it became evident to many surgeons that the procedure was adequate for advanced disease in the neck but was too aggressive for early N stages. Thus, to avoid the unnecessary removal of some neck structures, several conservation procedures were designed since the 1920s. This book will present the evolution of these "less than radical" operations from two different perspectives: the American and the Latin. The reason for this duality must be sought in the evolution of neck dissection. Over the years, this surgery has experienced the influence of two simultaneous tendencies, separated only by a language factor. This factor has produced a misunderstanding of ideas leading to a mismatch between concepts and surgical techniques.

The concept of a functional approach to the neck, materialized in the so-called functional neck dissection, has not been fully apprehended in the English literature. As a result, a new original idea has been identified as just another technical modification, which is included in a vast classification as just one more item.

This book tries to differentiate between conceptual approaches and surgical techniques. The former constitute keystones in the evolution of scientific knowledge. The latter are only technical variations of a standard procedure, designed to solve the problem using the most effective approach. Functional neck dissection belongs to the first group because it reflects a new original approach to the problem of lymph node metastases in head and neck cancer. On the other hand, selective neck dissections should be included within the group of surgical techniques because they share with functional neck dissection the same rationale and indications. Selective neck dissections constitute only technical variations of the functional concept, designed to fit the operation to the patient on a more individualized basis. The problem of functional and selective neck dissection will thus be addressed in this book from a different, nonconventional perspective: functional refers to a concept, and selective refers to surgical techniques included within this concept.

However, we do not intend this book to be merely a summary of the history and philosophy of neck dissection. We would like to bring this book to the medical shelves, not to the libraries of history. Therefore, we provide a detailed description of the anatomical basis and surgical technique of the functional approach to the neck. And by "functional approach to the neck" we mean any type of neck dissection that uses the basic principles of fascial dissection. Fascial spaces and barriers of the neck hold the rationale for functional neck dissection. This idea will be repeatedly emphasized throughout the text.

Finally, we include a comprehensive list of technical hints and pitfalls that the authors have learned through the years. These details, along with the answers to the most frequently asked questions regarding functional neck dissection, complete the contents of this book and contribute to the book's general purpose.

What This Book Is Not About

Now that you know what this book is about, we would like to make a few comments on the things that you will not find in the following pages. This book does not contain a detailed description of the surgical technique for all types of selective neck dissection. This is precisely what we try to avoid in an effort to stop further misunderstanding of the problem. Because selective neck dissections are regarded as technical modifications to the functional approach, they are all included in the general operative description. The step-by-step description of the complete surgical technique of functional neck dissection contains all the modifications that may be designed to treat the neck in patients with primary tumors from different sites, as long as these modifications follow the same rationale and basic indications of the original procedure. By describing the complete basic operation, all variations are included. Only specific surgical details of different types of selective operations will be mentioned in the text.

This book does not include an exhaustive discussion about the indications and usefulness of different types of selective neck dissection. History has proved the oncological safety of the concept of functional neck dissection for head and neck cancer. The nodal metastatic pattern for different head and neck primary tumors is well known, and some selective neck dissections have also proved to be totally safe. However, reducing the field of surgery creates a greater potential risk for leaving metastatic nodes behind.

We cannot assure the oncological safety of all types of selective neck dissection on the basis of our own personal experience. Preserving some nodal groups in carefully selected patients has been demonstrated to be oncologically safe in our hands (e.g., not including area I in patients with cancer of the larynx). However, we have not sufficiently tested other selective operations. Thus, extensive discussion about the indications for different types of selective neck dissection according to the location of the primary tumor will not be included in this book.

Finally, this book does not intend to propose a new classification of neck dissection. Our purpose is to present the rationale, surgical technique, and evolution of "less than radical" neck dissection from a historical perspective, emphasizing a conceptual approach over technical considerations. We seek to connect and unify the American and Latin points of view and thereby to clarify the confused field of nonradical neck dissection.

1 The Historical Outlook of Neck Dissection

1.1 Crile and the Radical Neck Dissection

The "grandfather" of neck dissection is George Crile, Sr., of the Cleveland Clinic. In 1906, Crile portrayed the field of head-and-neck surgery as being behind the times in terms of interest and progress. Crile believed that, if the neck lymphatics could be removed in a "radical" manner and "en bloc," more cures could be accomplished. The oncological approach to the neck proposed by Crile was strongly influenced by the oncologic principles used by Halstead for breast cancer. The concept of the "bloc" that was in vogue for the treatment of breast cancer required removal of the primary site with draining lymphatics and nodes in continuity. In breast surgery, the pectoralis muscle and the axillary vein were part of the "bloc," as were all other structures surrounding the tumor. No oncological benefits beyond access were claimed.

Following these principles, Crile designed a similar operation to remove the lymphatic system of the neck in patients with head-and-neck tumors. Here, the sternocleidomastoid muscle and the internal jugular vein suffered the same fate as the pectoralis muscle and the axillary vein in breast cancer surgery. Crile's procedure allowed a systematic removal of the lymphatic tissue of the neck, along with the surrounding structures. Only the carotid artery and some "lucky" nerves survived the Halstedian concept of oncological surgery. This operation received the name of "Radical Neck Dissection" and was popularized by Hayes Martin.

The work of Martin completely changed the world of neck dissection. Radical neck dissection became the standard procedure for patients requiring surgical treatment of the lymphatics of the neck in combination with removal of the primary tumor. The lymphatic tissue had to be removed from the neck and the best way to do this was by removing almost every single structure within the cervical area.

1.2 Time to Change

The analogous thinking between general surgery and head-and-neck surgery persisted until the early 1960s when general surgeons began to reconsider the usefulness of the "*bigger is better*" concept in breast cancer. Head-and-neck surgeons had a similar evolution. It was evident to all those involved in the management of patients with head-and-neck cancer that the radical operation was adequate for the treatment of large palpable masses. But two new issues gained importance in the field of head-and-neck cancer surgery: the need for treatment of the N0 neck, and the need for simultaneous bilateral neck dissection.

The need to treat the neck in patients without palpable disease became evident at the light of the knowledge of the biological behavior of the lymphatic metastases. Some primary tumors were associated with a high rate of false clinical and radiological N0 necks, leading to a high incidence of neck recurrences that could be prevented by neck dissection. The radical operation was considered too aggressive for these patients. The concept "elective neck dissection" became soon a matter of debate. Some authors refer to elective neck dissection as prophylactic neck dissection. This is a clear misuse of the term "*prophylactic*." Prophylaxis implies prevention of something to happen. In Martin's time, there was the subtle suggestion that a prophylactic dissection actually prevented something, but what that something was is not clear. Neck dissection does not prevent either neck relapse or anything: it either treats existing neck metastases (evident or occult) or provides valuable information about the actual absence of metastases. Nowadays, the concept of *prophylactic* neck dissection is clearly faulty. From an oncologic standpoint, a neck dissection is either therapeutic, when positive nodes are found in the specimen, or oncologically useless, when positive nodes are not identified in the surgical specimen. However, there are other nononcological advantages of neck dissection. Namely, prognostic information—a true N0 patient has around 50% more chances of survival than an N+ patient—and postoperative treatment planning.

Another argument in favor of less aggressive neck dissections was the possibility of bilateral neck metastasis that some head-and-neck tumors have. Multiple studies about cervical lymph flow demonstrated that head-and-neck midline structures could metastasize with similar probabilities to both sides of the neck. It was noteworthy that radical neck dissection was not practical as a simultaneous bilateral procedure. The need for less aggressive types of neck dissection became evident also in these cases.

1.2.1 Changing the Paradigm

Changes in life can be made using two different approaches: modifying what needs to be changed, or creating something new to replace the old element. The end result may look similar—something new taking over the place of the old concept—but the approach to change is radically different.

There is an easy example of what we try to explain. Imagine you live in the 1960s and have one of these big black telephones at home with a large dial full of numbers. Now, you want to create a new telephone that you can take with you in your pocket. You can modify what you have at home and design a small device with a keypad that

1

can be used to talk to distant people. Nokia did that for you. That was a modification of the classic telephone. Now, imagine that you design something different. Something that has a camera, can play music, has an agenda, connects to internet, allows you to pay, and you move items on the screen by touching them with your fingers. Steve Jobs did this. And this is, by no means, a modification of the old phone we had at home. This is a completely new idea.

The same happened with neck dissection. In the United States, the old radical neck dissection was modified to make it less aggressive. In some Latin countries (Argentina, Spain, Italy) a new way to approach the neck was designed. It was called "functional neck dissection," and it was not a modified radical neck dissection. It was a completely new way to remove the lymphatic tissue of the neck.

1.3 Modified Radical Neck Dissection

From Martin's time, surgeons recognized that the Crile operation was not always necessary and was unwarranted in some cases of head-and-neck cancer. Data assured surgeons that neck recurrence rates with pathologically negative necks and low-staged clinically positive necks were similar regardless whether the accessory nerve was sacrificed or not. The long-term functional consequences of accessory nerve sacrifice were described in the 1960s as the shoulder syndrome. Shoulder droop, diminished range of motion, shoulder abduction, and external rotation and pain led to reconsideration of routine nerve sacrifice. Modified neck dissection that preserved the accessory nerve was a logical first modification. It later became obvious that preserving the nerve, by dissecting it free, was not always followed by normal nerve function. Surgical trauma during dissection left some with variations of the shoulder syndrome. Questionnaires about shoulder function were reassuring but electromyography and careful clinical evaluation by experts documented that preserving the accessory nerve is not always enough. However, careful nerve preservation is more rational than routine sacrifice of the nerve.

The loss of contour after removal of the sternocleidomastoid muscle led also to reconsideration of that practice. The muscle does not contain lymphatics or lymph nodes, but its removal does make neck dissection easier. Routine sacrifice of the jugular vein adds no oncological safety in the clinically negative and low-stage clinically positive neck situations. For surgeons who favored elective and bilateral dissections, it was evident that the radical operation was excessive when no metastases were found in the neck.

The team at UT MD Anderson Cancer Center, including Richard H. Jesse and Alando J. Ballantyne, pioneered modified neck dissections in the United States, and they first reported their results in the American Journal of Surgery in an article titled "Radical or modified neck dissection: a therapeutic dilemma" in 1978. Soon surgeons in the United States accepted that "less than radical neck dissection" was a good option in selected patients and the terms *modified, supraomohyoid, upper, midline* were used to describe these lesser operations.

The nomenclature became confusing to teach and lacked standardization for reporting. The American Academy of Otolaryngology—Head and Neck Surgery convened a special task force to address the terminology problems. The group was tasked to (1) recommend terminology that adhered to the more traditional words as radical and modified radical; (2) define which lymphatic structures and other nonlymphatic structures would be removed relative to the radical dissection; (3) provide a standard nomenclature for lymph node groups and nonlymphatic structures; (4) define the boundaries for resection of lymph node groups; (5) use terms for neck dissection procedures that are basic and easy to understand; and (6) develop a classification based on the biology of cervical metastases and the principles of oncological surgery.

Some of these goals were accomplished. Terminology was fashioned, and lymph node groups were defined, as were the boundaries of the groups. Whether these accomplishments created a system, basic and easy to use, is in doubt. The Academy classification was based on the rationale that (1) radical neck dissection is the standard reference procedure; (2) when one or more nonlymphoid structures are preserved, the term *modified neck dissection* is preferred; (3) when one or more lymphoid groups are preserved, the term *selective dissection* is recommended; and (4) when a procedure removes other lymph node groups or nonlymphoid structures different from those removed in the radical neck dissection, the recommended term is *extended neck dissection*.

The Academy classification defined seven different neck dissections (▶ Table 1.1). Other classifications are cited in the literature and preferred by their authors' institutions, so the classification issue is not unanimously agreed upon. For example, Spiro from Memorial Hospital offers a list of 11 neck dissections (▶ Table 1.2). Medina modified the Academy classification with eight different types of comprehensive neck dissection, seven selective operations,

Table 1.1 The American Academy of Otolaryngology—head-and-neck surgery classification of neck dissection

Radical neck dissection
Modified radical neck dissection
Selective neck dissection
Supraomohyoid neck dissection
Lateral neck dissection
Posterolateral neck dissection
Anterior neck dissection
Extended neck dissection

Table 1.2 Memorial Hospital Classification of neck dissection proposed by Spiro

Radical (four or five node levels)
Conventional radical
Modified radical
Extended radical
Modified and extended radical
Selective (three node levels)
Supraomohyoid
Jugular neck dissection
Any other three node level dissection
Limited neck dissection
Posterolateral
Paratracheal
Mediastinal
Any other one or two node levels

Table 1.3 Medina's modification of the American Academy Classification of neck dissection

Comprehensive	Selective
Radical	Lateral
Subtype A	Anterolateral
Subtype B	Supraomohyoid
Modified radical	Posterolateral
Type IA	Radical
Type IB	Type I
Type IIA	Type II
Type IIB	Type III
Type IIIA	Extended
Type IIIB	

and one extended neck dissection (▶ Table 1.3). A classification published in 2011 by several renowned authors attempting a consensus proposed that the symbol "ND" be followed by the lymphatic levels removed and nonlymphatic structures resected. In our opinion, all these proposals add very little to clarifying the field of neck dissection from a practical educational standpoint.

What is not clear, on a statistically supported basis, is what dissection is appropriate for what clinical scenario. The question of whether many of the modifications make any clinical difference, in terms of survival, morbidity, or any other measure of value recognized today, has not been answered. Only empirical assumption is offered as a basis for these recommendations. It is unlikely that statistical data will be forthcoming in the immediate future because the whole issue of the type of neck dissection is being overshadowed by the questions raised about neck treatment when concomitant chemoradiotherapy programs are used as initial treatment for both the primary site and neck metastases.

Names like Robert M. Byers, Eugene N. Myers, Lawrence W. DeSanto, Jonas T. Johnson, and many others were early adapters of modified radical neck dissection and published their results in several seminal articles in the mid-1990s.

1.3.1 Indications for Modified Neck Dissections

The classical radical neck dissection is too much for the patient with no clinical evidence of neck metastases. Moreover, it is not always successful with advanced metastatic disease (N2 and N3). Modifications recognize that what we do to patients may be less important than what patients bring to treatment with their immune systems. The human immune system plays a role in who gets well, the likelihood of recurrences in the neck, and the probability of a cure. Neck recurrences happen regardless of how radical or conservative the operation.

Radical neck dissection removes all the lymph node groups from the mandible to the clavicle, and from the midline of the neck to the anterior border of the trapezius muscle. Also, it removes the nodes in the tail of the parotid, the internal jugular vein, the spinal accessory nerve, and the sternomastoid muscle. The postauricular, suboccipital, buccinator, perifacial, and retropharyngeal nodes are not removed. The radical operation is recommended for extensive lymph node metastases, gross extranodal spread from nodal metastases, and lymph node metastases around the accessory nerve and internal jugular vein. It is the operation often used for surgical salvage after chemotherapy or radiation failure, for the previously violated neck, and for other difficult or indeterminate situations.

According to the classification of the American Academy of Otolaryngology—Head and Neck Surgery, modified radical neck dissection is the "en bloc" removal of the same lymph nodes and lymphatics as the radical operation (levels I to V) but with the preservation of one or more nonlymphatic structures routinely taken with the radical operation. The goal of modification is to lessen the morbidity resulting from the sacrifice of the accessory nerve. The morbidity of the removal of the internal jugular vein becomes an issue only when bilateral operations are performed. Preservation of the sternomastoid muscle is said to provide a cosmetic benefit.

The modified radical operation is indicated when an operation is needed to remove all gross nodal metastases while preserving the accessory nerve. This is possible when the metastatic disease is in no greater proximity to that nerve than it is to the vagus or hypoglossal nerves. These nerves were ritualistically preserved with the radical operation, whereas the accessory nerve was sacrificed.

1.3.2 Clinically Negative Neck

Martin's bias against elective (misnamed as prophylactic neck dissection, because no neck dissection is prophylactic) has been reexamined. Retrospective studies, reviews, and analyses suggest that watchful waiting after primary tumor treatment increases the risk of failure because of undetected disease in the neck. Risk varies with the site of the primary tumor. The probability of nonclinical or so-called occult metastases varies by the site and size of the primary tumor, as well as other variables such as depth of mucosal invasion of the primary tumor. Clinicians estimate these risks by palpation, imaging studies, and needle biopsies. The probability estimates are then used to attempt rational decisions on whether, when, and how to treat the clinically negative neck.

A growth in popularity of electively treating the neck has been the major stimulus to more conservative neck dissections. There is acknowledgment that many elective dissections do not remove any metastases because the neck nodes are truly negative. There is historical evidence that an operation less extensive than the radical neck dissection is just as effective in controlling occult metastases. A new philosophy is evolving. That philosophy asks, *What unnecessary treatment is least harmful?* not, *What necessary treatment is most effective? Necessary* refers to when disease is present and *unnecessary* to when it is not. Shah, for example, found that two-thirds of patients undergoing elective neck dissection did not have metastatic cancer. Less radical surgery nurtures a selective approach to surgical neck treatment.

Evaluation of the clinically negative neck is now more dependent on technology than it was in the past. Clinical evaluation by palpation is essential but unreliable in detecting so-called occult, microscopic, or subclinical lymph node metastases. Word confusion also influences treatment planning. *Occult* or *subclinical* means not palpable and uncertain with imaging studies. *Microscopic* means disease that can only be detected with the microscopic examination of a removed specimen. These distinctions are important to the issue of radiation treatment to the neck of the patient without evidence of metastases.

Palpation is said to be in error 20 to 50% of the time. Accuracy depends on the examiner's experience, the patient's physical habitus (e.g., short fat necks vs. thin long necks), prior neck treatment (including open neck biopsy), and prior radiotherapy to the neck. Recent advances in imaging techniques with computed tomography (CT), magnetic resonance (MR), ultrasound and PET-CT scans have decreased the error rate in staging the necks when small cancer-containing nodes cannot be palpated. Criteria for malignancy on CT and MR include (1) nodal size of 15 mm or more in level II and 10 mm in other levels; (2) groups of three or more questionable nodes 1 to 2 mm smaller; (3) nodes of any size with central necrosis; and (4) loss of tissue (i.e., fat) planes within imaged nodes. These criteria are fallible and continue to be refined. Size is the least reliable criteria. Using the > 10 mm threshold, Friedman et al found a sensitivity of 95% but a specificity of only 77%. Using > 15 mm as the threshold, Feinmesser

et al found a sensitivity of only 60% and a specificity of 85%. Central lucency can be misleading. It can be caused by fat in the node or an artery with plaque formation. Fine needle aspiration, guided by ultrasound, improves accuracy in diagnosis that approaches 90% when carried out by experts in both ultrasound and fine needle biopsy. PET-CT has a high sensitivity, but lacks specificity.

In practice, the decision to electively treat the neck of a patient with a clinically negative neck is made on the clinical assessment of the primary site, an estimate of probability of metastases, and the uncertain support from imaging studies.

1.3.3 Selective Neck Dissection

The MD Anderson University of Texas Cancer Center and the Memorial Sloan-Kettering group popularized the concept of selective neck dissection.

Lymph Node Groups

The concept of radical and modified radical neck dissection considers the cervical lymph nodes as a unified system divided into anatomical areas such as upper, lower, posterior, and submandibular. The selective dissection movement in the United States focuses more on the subgroups than the system as a whole. The selective dissection model uses retrospective studies that support the idea that metastases from the various sites in the head and neck have predictable patterns in early stages. The movement is a logical outgrowth of the concept of conservation surgery and a movement away from the "more is better" philosophy.

The most popular terminology for subdividing the lymph node groups is that used by the head-and-neck surgery department at the Memorial Sloan-Kettering Hospital. This classification divides the neck into five levels in each side of the neck. A sixth zone describes the anterior compartments of the neck. A complete description of level and boundaries of lymph node groups is provided in the next chapter.

Using the Selective Neck Dissections

The idea of selective neck dissection appears to have started for neck management of lip cancer at the MD Anderson Hospital. Jesse and Fletcher raised the question of radical versus modified radical neck dissection in 1978. At the Mayo Clinic, surgeons were performing a modified neck dissection with preservation of the accessory nerve from the early 1960s when Ward et al reported on this modification.

Selective neck dissections are used on patients with known limited disease or a probability of limited disease. The operations are based on the predictability of metastatic patterns depending on the primary site. Level or levels of nodes removed depend on the location of the primary tumor. Selectivity in neck dissection depends on the principle that, in the early stages, metastatic patterns are predictable in previously untreated cancers.

Information concerning the metastatic pattern from different head-and-neck primary sites has allowed a more selective type of neck dissection. The issue is why? The removal of nonlymphatic structures causes the morbidity of neck dissection. One can question the rationale for saving proximate nodal groups that merge into one another. In the United States, the concept of selective neck dissection is popular, but difficult to use. Selective dissections are recommended only for early and previously untreated cancer. With the popularity of so-called organ preservation programs in clinical studies and the community, the treatment of previously untreated cancers by the surgeon is not as common as when the concept of selective neck dissection was evolving.

Selective Neck Dissection: Final Issues

A surgeon from somewhere other than the United States might wonder what purpose is served by trying to classify what surgeons have always done. The importance may be more nononcological than oncological. We perceive the selective classification's role as part of the medical reimbursement system of the United States. Insurance companies and government health care funding systems prefer categorical descriptions of what they are paying for by codifying selective procedures as much as is possible. This motive is seldom stated. There are unanticipated consequences of this manipulation of the nomenclature. Major cancer center guidelines separate the head-and-neck oncological specialists in the community from those in the cancer centers. This may have been an unstated goal rather than an unintended consequence. With seven or more primary sites, four primary stages, three or more neck disease stages, seven or more kinds of neck dissections, and two sides of the neck, the practitioner has to choose among so many permutations and combinations that the neck may be undertreated, overtreated, or not treated at all. Out of frustration, the patient may be referred to the medical center. The experienced surgeon may well be comfortable with intuitively picking and choosing among options. The community surgeon, who is less comfortable with so many options, may give up, and refer away, radiate the neck, or not treat the neck nodes in the elective situation. As educators who listened to more than one hundred resident physicians discuss their ideas about proper neck treatment strategies, we have perceived their confusion. An experienced surgeon can use selective neck dissections in selected situations. The decision is usually intuitive and based on the conviction that bilateral neck dissections are at times important. Martin's caution remains about the absence of infallibility and the certainty that there are no reliable statistical data to support many of these decisions. The whole concept of selective neck dissection may well be rendered moot in the

United States because so much more surgery for neck metastases is being done after chemoradiotherapy either in a planned sequence in advanced (N2 and N3) neck metastatic disease or in the salvage at recurrence after chemoradiotherapy failure.

1.4 Functional Neck Dissection

In 1968, César Gavilán, at that time Chairman of the Department of Otorhinolaryngology at La Paz University Hospital in Madrid, Spain, was invited to lecture on vestibular disorders at the Medical School of the University of Córdoba (Argentina). Osvaldo Suárez was among the attendants (► Fig. 1.1). Although Suárez was employed in the Department of Otolaryngology, he also worked at the Department of Anatomy under the direction of Pedro Ara. Professor Ara was known in Argentina as the "Spanish anatomist," and he was very popular for having embalmed the corpse of Eva Perón (► Fig. 1.2). The dual projection of

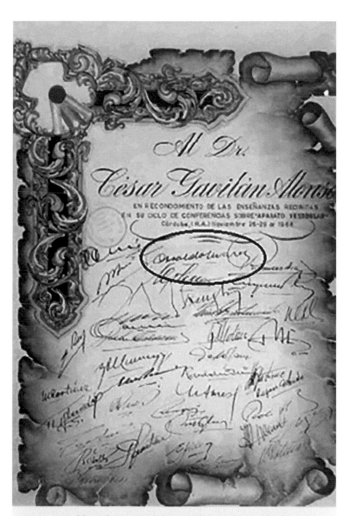

Fig. 1.1 Osvaldo Suárez signed this certificate, along with the remaining attendants, in recognition of the course on vestibular disorders given by C. Gavilán, MD, in Córdoba, Argentina (November 1968).

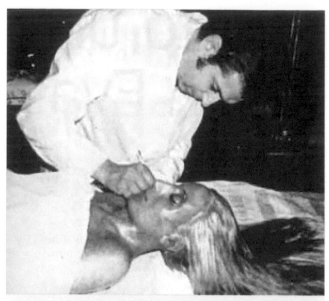

Fig. 1.2 Professor Pedro Ara ("The Spanish Anatomist") embalming the corpse of Eva Perón in 1952.

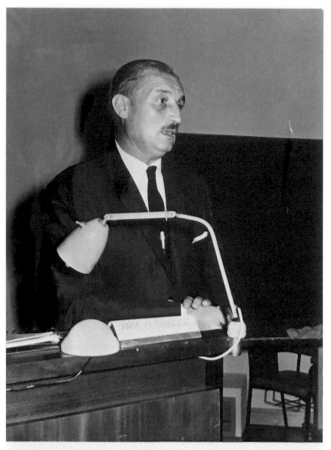

Fig. 1.3 Osvaldo Suárez during one of his lectures at La Paz Hospital in Madrid (June 1969).

Suárez as anatomist and otolaryngologist conferred a privileged position on him. On the one hand, as otolaryngologist he had a thorough knowledge of head-and-neck cancer—especially cancer of the larynx. On the other, as anatomist he was very familiar with all anatomical details concerning neck dissection.

After the course, Suárez approached César Gavilán and invited him to watch a couple of surgical cases of cancer of the larynx with their respective functional neck dissections. *This is a new approach to the neck that I have developed for N0 patients and patients with small nodes not fixed to surrounding structures*, he said. The next morning, they both went to the operating room. César Gavilán was shocked with what he saw. The experience was striking—truly an instance of fortune knocking at his door. The operation, as performed by Suárez, was nothing like he had seen before. It was clean, systematic, comprehensive, and easy to understand and teach. Moreover, it looked extremely useful from an oncologic standpoint.

As a consequence, he immediately arranged for Suárez to visit Madrid in the coming year to stay at La Paz University Hospital for 2 weeks. During the first week he would perform as many operations as possible with the team of the Department. The second week would be devoted to a course on cancer of the larynx. He accepted the invitation.

In spite of his subsequently being diagnosed with a serious disease—hypernephroma—he attended to his date in Madrid. In June 1969, he spent a week operating daily on head-and-neck cancer patients in the Department of Otorhinolaryngology, La Paz University Hospital, Madrid, Spain. A second week was dedicated to teaching Functional Neck Dissection during a course in which he alternated lectures with live surgery demonstrations (▶ Fig. 1.3).

An arrangement was made to bring him back again to Madrid to repeat the exciting experience, but, unfortunately, the political situation in Argentina became difficult, with the military dictatorship taking over the country. The dark days of the Argentinian history prevented Osvaldo Suárez from coming back to Madrid.

In 1972 while he was at home watching the news on TV, the speaker mentioned that a young lady had been killed by the military during a shooting on the streets. Osvaldo Suárez died from a heart attack. That young lady was his daughter... Some years after this sad episode, another of his sons disappeared on one of those miserable flights over the sea where people were thrown alive into the ocean. His 99-year-old widow is still alive when these pages are being written.

1.4.1 The Origins of Functional Neck Dissection

"If you think you have discovered something new, it is because you do not read enough." This popular statement summarizes the philosophy of most innovations in the field of science. The great contributions to human knowledge are always the result of a combination of previous research and personal experience. However, almost every important scientific discovery is linked to a person's name. Functional neck dissection must be associated with the name and the person of Osvaldo Suárez.

It is true that from the very beginning it became evident to many that radical neck dissection was too aggressive in a large number of situations. Some surgeons like Truffert, Silvester Begnis, and others tried to modify what was considered to be the standard approach at that time, but their attempts were not fully successful. However, they laid the foundations on which future developments could be built. Osvaldo Suárez must be credited as the person responsible for gathering the previous knowledge with his own experience—oncological and anatomical—into a new approach for the management of neck metastasis in patients with head-and-neck cancer. The result of this combination of background, experience, and surgical ability was called functional neck dissection.

Two different factors should be considered on functional neck dissection: (1) the spirit of the procedure; and (2) its surgical technique.

The Spirit of Functional Neck Dissection

The main goal of the "functional" approach to neck dissection proposed by Suárez is the removal of all lymphatic tissue in the neck, preserving the remaining neck structures. This is achieved by using the fascial planes of the neck that surround most cervical structures and separate them from the adjacent lymphatic tissue (see Chapter 2 of this book).

As long as the tumor cells remain confined within the lymphatic system of the neck, they can be safely removed by carefully stripping the neck structures from their fascial covering. There is no oncological benefit from removing the sternocleidomastoid muscle, internal jugular vein, or any other important neck structure, when cancer is locked up inside a partially isolated lymphatic space. The situation changes when the lesion invades the walls of this anatomical container, fixing the nodes to surrounding structures. Then, the tumor is no longer a "nodal cancer" but becomes a "neck cancer." This situation invalidates the "functional" spirit and justifies the use of a classic approach with removal of the involved neck structures.

Therefore, the spirit of functional neck dissection is to take advantage of the particular anatomy of the neck to remove **all** or **part of** the lymphatic system, with preservation of the remaining neck structures. The key words in this definition are **all** and **part of**. The spirit of functional neck dissection does not take into consideration the extension of the removal. Functional neck dissection only intends to use the fascial planes of the neck to carry the desired removal without disturbing the surrounding structures. It may include all the lymphatic tissue of the neck—all nodal regions—or only some selected groups, according to the expected incidence of cervical metastasis,

the location and extent of the primary tumor, and the preferences of the surgeon. When the operation was adopted by American surgeons, these important words vanished, and the concept of functional neck dissection—the spirit of the procedure—was seriously affected.

For supraglottic cancer, Osvaldo Suárez never included in the resection the submental and submandibular lymph nodes (area I). Obviously, he also did not include the central compartment of the neck (area VI) for these lesions. However, he still considered this to be a functional neck dissection, as long as the main principle of dissecting through fascial planes was guiding the surgeon's hands.

It may be argued that preservation of some nodal groups requires cutting through the fibrofatty tissue that contains the lymphatic system of the neck, something that seems to be in contradiction with the basic principle of fascial dissection. This is only a theoretical concern with no practical implications, as has been proved by the results of the functional approach over the years. In fact, it must be remembered that nodal groups are only a schematic representation of the lymphatic system of the neck, which is really configured in different chains that follow the course of the major cervical vessels and nerves (see Chapter 2). Modified radical neck dissection with spinal accessory nerve preservation also requires sectioning the lymphatic container in the upper part of the neck to preserve the anatomical integrity of the nerve between the jugular foramen and the sternocleidomastoid muscle. The theoretical drawbacks of this maneuver—cutting through lymphatic tissue and violating fascial barriers—have never been a problem with respect to oncological results, as long as its indications are carefully observed.

To summarize, the spirit of functional neck dissection may be compared with the philosophy of partial laryngectomy. Total laryngectomy goes against the organ and removes the whole larynx with the tumor that it contains, whereas partial laryngectomy is directed against the tumor and preserves the functioning part of the larynx that is not involved by the tumor. Both approaches have their own rationale, role, and indications, and neither can be considered to be a modification of the other. The same can be said of functional and radical neck dissection.

Surgical Technique of Functional Neck Dissection

We give special emphasis to the difference between the spirit (i.e., functional neck dissection as a concept) and the surgical technique (i.e., just one more operation). As a surgeon one can apply the spirit without the surgical technique and vice versa.

The technical details of the functional approach play a secondary role for the understanding of the procedure, although they have been given a major interest. Factors such as the extension of the operation, its technical difficulty, the time required to perform the procedure, and others have been the center of debate for many years. It is true that most of them deserve some attention, but, obviously, they are not the main issue.

Concerns about the extension of the operation have been discussed previously and will be emphasized in other chapters of this book. Technical difficulty is a relative problem. For those, like us, who have been trained in this operation since the very beginning of our professional careers, functional neck dissection is much easier than the classic radical operation. Why? Simply because we have performed many more functional operations than radical procedures. This demonstrates the relativity of the issue of difficulty. The same can be said about the idea of functional neck dissection as a time-consuming operation. Obviously, for the N0 neck it will take more time to perform a complete functional neck dissection than a radical operation. However, the time difference will also depend on the experience of the surgeon, and, again, those familiar with the functional operation will find the difference to be less important. This is not to mention the cosmetic, anatomical, and functional disadvantages of performing radical neck dissections in N0 necks—something that very few appropriately trained surgeons will still support today.

Another technical factor that Osvaldo Suárez usually emphasized was the type of dissection performed (e.g., knife vs. blunt dissection). As an anatomist, he stressed the advantage of knife dissection over blunt dissection to follow the fascial planes of the neck. Some of us learned his lesson and still use the scalpel for most of the surgical steps in functional neck dissection. The technical details for a successful knife dissection along with some practical tips are given in the following chapters.

The Functional Approach: Combination of Spirit and Technique

Applying the technical details of functional neck dissection without understanding the spirit of the procedure results in a large number of different operations, be they selective operations, modified procedures, limited neck dissections, or any other name we would like to use. This is in part what happens with most neck dissection classifications currently used in the literature. On the other hand, understanding the spirit of the procedure but using wrong technical abilities produces a messy operation that is difficult to understand and teach. The operation will not look appealing and the observer will have a bad feeling about it.

As for any other human activity, approaching perfection requires a balanced combination of ideas and skills. This is achieved only by putting together the technical details with the spirit of the procedure. This is what we call functional neck dissection.

1.4.2 Evolution of Functional Neck Dissection

Osvaldo Suárez did a fine job with functional neck dissection. He had a thorough knowledge of neck anatomy, was a great surgeon, and designed a new approach to the lymphatic system of the neck for patients with head-and-neck cancer. He was also able to teach the operation to those avid surgeons desiring to assist or observe him at surgery. However, he had an important weak point: he did not dedicate enough time to promote the diffusion of his technique within the scientific community. In fact, he published only a couple of papers that were indirectly related to functional neck dissection. In his most frequently cited paper, "El problema de las metástasis linfáticas y alejadas del cáncer de laringe e hipofaringe," he describes the anatomical basis for functional neck dissection, without an in-depth description of the surgical technique.

1.4.3 Functional Neck Dissection after Osvaldo Suárez

In his last years Suárez taught the procedure to two prominent disciples. Both were especially interested in the operation for patients with cancer of the larynx because both were otolaryngologists in Latin countries where there is an extremely high incidence of cancer of the larynx—especially supraglottic lesions. The incidence of bilateral neck metastasis in these lesions, along with the need to treat N0 patients, made functional neck dissection the ideal tool for this group of patients. The names of these enthusiastic pupils were César Gavilán, from Spain, and Ettore Bocca, from Italy. They both learned the operation directly from Suárez. They both understood that this could be the solution to their problems with N0 patients and bilateral neck dissections, and they both adopted functional neck dissection as a new revolutionary approach to the neck. Suárez also left a well-trained disciple, who was his relative, Dr. Filiberti, but he died shortly thereafter, taking with him the knowledge and the tradition of Suárez's experience in Argentina.

César Gavilán introduced functional neck dissection in Spain in the late 1960s and early 1970s. Ettore Bocca did the same in Italy. However, Bocca also published his results in the English literature. This explains the common association of functional neck dissection with Bocca's name so often found in the Anglo-Saxon countries. However, if one reads carefully Bocca's papers on functional neck dissection, the name of Suárez is always mentioned.

Functional neck dissection arrived in the United States more than a decade after it was introduced in Europe, but, more important, it did so through the experience and words of third parties. Thus, part of the message vanished in the process of adaptation to the new environment. Unfortunately, the part missing was the philosophical element of the message, supposedly the less important piece of information—in reality, the core of the new procedure.

In the United States, the operation soon became accepted as an oncologically safe procedure for the management of the neck in head-and-neck cancer patients.

However, it was considered just a simple modification of the classic procedure described by Crile and was included as one more item in a vast classification of different types of neck dissection. The surgical technique was there, but the concept—the spirit of the procedure—did not reach the head-and-neck surgeons in the United States.

The real concept of functional neck dissection was lost in translation!

2 The Rationale and Anatomical Basis for Functional and Selective Neck Dissection

2.1 Introduction

Functional neck dissection, as described by Osvaldo Suárez, is based on the existence of a fascial barrier between the lymphatic tissue and the muscular, glandular, neural, and vascular structures of the neck. This anatomical separation allows the creation of a surgical plane of dissection. The fascial layer invests muscles and organs in the neck, forming planes and spaces where many important structures are crowded together. This fact, known as fascial compartmentalization, holds the rationale for functional neck dissection.

This chapter describes the anatomical bases of functional neck dissection from a practical and surgical standpoint.

2.2 Rationale for Functional and Selective Neck Dissection

2.2.1 Fascial Anatomy of the Neck

The anatomical description of the fascial layers of the neck has suffered a number of different descriptions. For practical reasons we will consider two distinct fascial layers in the neck, the superficial cervical fascia and the deep cervical fascia. The superficial cervical fascia corresponds to the subcutaneous tissue. The deep cervical fascia is the key element for functional and selective neck dissection.

The *superficial cervical fascia* extends from the zygoma down to the clavicle, enveloping the platysma muscle and the muscles of facial expression. The vascularization of the skin forms a net superficial to the platysma muscle, within the superficial cervical fascia, with few branches connecting this net to the underlying vascular supply. There is a potential space between the superficial fascia and the deep fascia that allows free movement of the skin and superficial fascia on deeper structures. This plane, located underneath the platysma muscle, is the cleavage plane that should be followed to properly elevate the cutaneous flaps in functional and selective neck dissection as well as other surgical procedures in the neck. By elevating the cutaneous flaps on this plane, the net that vascularize the skin is preserved, while the dissection is carried out on a relatively avascular plane (► Fig. 2.1).

The *deep cervical fascia* (► Fig. 2.2) surrounds the neck, enveloping its different structures. For teaching purposes,

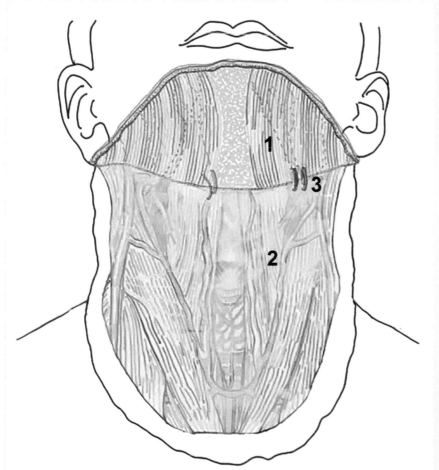

Fig. 2.1 Schematic view of the neck after raising the skin flaps. The vascular net within the superficial cervical fascia is represented by transparency of the platysma muscle. Some vessels anastomose this net with the underlying vasculature, crossing the platysma muscle and the superficial layer of the deep cervical fascia. These later vessels should be coagulated during the dissection of the skin flaps. 1, superior skin flap; 2, superficial layer of the deep cervical fascia; 3, anastomosing vessels.

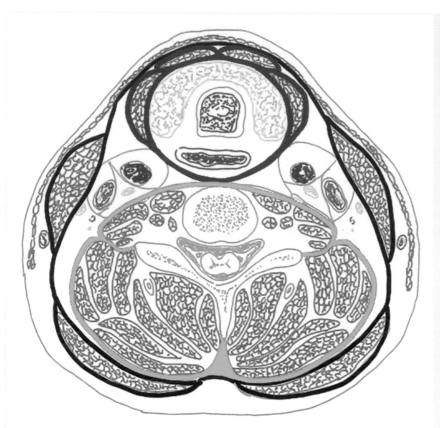

Fig. 2.2 Horizontal cross-section of the neck at the level of the sixth cervical vertebra showing the three layers of the deep cervical fascia: superficial layer (black color), middle or visceral layer (purple color), and deep or prevertebral layer (green color).

three different layers are considered within the deep cervical fascia: a superficial, a middle, and a deep or prevertebral layer. The carotid sheath, which is an important structure from the surgical standpoint, is located between these layers of the deep cervical fascia.

The *superficial layer* of the deep cervical fascia, also known as investing or anterior fascia, completely envelops the neck with the exception of the skin, platysma muscle, and superficial fascia. Superiorly, it is attached to the occipital protuberance, mastoid process, capsule of the parotid gland, and body of the mandible. As it descends, it passes anteriorly from the mandible to the hyoid bone and from here down to the sternum, and posteriorly it passes across the spinal processes of the cervical vertebrae and the ligamentum nuchae. Inferiorly, it attaches to the sternum, upper edge of the clavicle, acromion, and spine of the scapula. At the inferior border, in the midline, the superficial layer splits in two different layers just superior to the manubrium of the sternum, enclosing the *suprasternal space of Burns*. From posterior to anterior, the superficial layer splits to enclose the trapezius, the inferior body of the omohyoid muscle as it crosses the posterior triangle of the neck, and the sternocleidomastoid muscle. The superficial veins of the neck lie on or within this superficial layer of the deep cervical fascia.

The *middle layer,* or *visceral layer,* envelops the upper aerodigestive tract. Superiorly, it is known as *buccopharyngeal fascia,* which inserts in the skull base and surrounds the posterior and lateral aspects of the nasopharynx and the oropharynx. Further down, the visceral layer is attached to the hyoid bone and encircles the strap muscles (except for the inferior body of the omohyoid muscle), the larynx and the trachea along with the hypopharynx and the esophagus. The thyroid and the parathyroid glands, as well as the recurrent laryngeal nerves and the central compartment lymph nodes are also surrounded by the visceral layer. Inferiorly, it merges with the pericardium inside the mediastinum.

The *deep* or *prevertebral layer* encloses the vertebral column and the paraspinal and prevertebral muscles. It attaches posteriorly to the spinous processes of the cervical vertebrae and ligamentum nuchae, and laterally to the anterior tubercles of the transverse process of the cervical vertebrae. At its superior limit, it goes to the skull base at the jugular foramen and carotid canal, then passes across the basilar process to the opposite side. In the upper part of the neck, this fascial layer covers the muscles of the back that enter into the lateral neck immediately deep to the trapezius muscle (splenius and levator scapula). At this level, there is a potential space between superficial and deep layers that is crossed by the spinal accessory nerve,

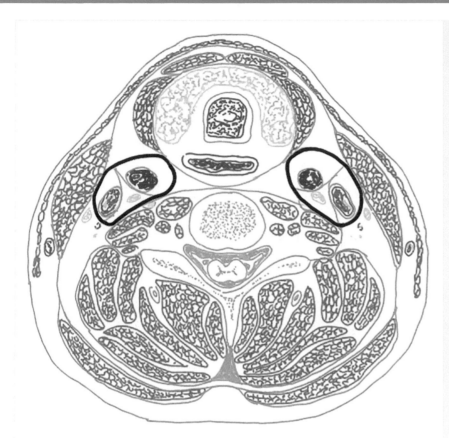

Fig. 2.3 Horizontal cross-section of the neck at the level of the sixth cervical vertebra showing the carotid sheath. Note that it is composed by contributions of the three layers of the deep cervical fascia.

along with some lymph nodes. At the lower end, both fascial layers further separate, the deep layer covering the scalene muscles, whereas the superficial layer remains attached to the trapezius muscle and the clavicle. The phrenic nerve runs inferiorly on the anterior aspect of the scalene group, covered by the deep fascial layer.

The *carotid sheath* or *vascular sheath* lies between the different layers of the deep cervical fascia and is composed by contributions of the three of them (▶ Fig. 2.3). This vascular sheath runs from the base of the skull to the root of the neck. It may be regarded as a cylinder-like structure with independent compartments for the internal jugular vein, the carotid artery, the vagus nerve, and the ansa cervicalis. The cervical portion of the sympathetic trunk runs posterior to the carotid sheath, within the prevertebral layer.

Fascial compartmentalization allows the removal of cervical lymphatic tissue by separating and removing the fascial walls of these "containers" along with their contents from the underlying vascular, glandular, neural, and muscular structures.

2.2.2 Lymph Node Distribution: Lymphatic Chains

The lymphatic system of the neck consists of a network of lymph nodes intimately connected by lymphatic channels.

For teaching purposes, two major lymphatic networks may be considered in the neck, a superficial and a deep web.

Superficial Lymphatics

The superficial lymphatics of the head and neck drain the skin into the superficial lymph nodes located around the neck and along the external and anterior jugular veins. Superficial lymphatics include the submental, submandibular, external jugular, anterior jugular, occipital, mastoid, and parotid groups (▶ Fig. 2.4).

The *submental nodes*, usually two or three in number, lie in a midline triangular space bounded by the anterior bellies of the digastric muscles and the hyoid bone. They drain the skin of the chin, the skin and mucous membrane of the central portion of the lower lip and jaw, the floor of the mouth, and the tip of the tongue. These nodes drain into the submandibular chain or directly into the deep cervical chains.

The *submandibular nodes* are located along the inferior border of the horizontal ramus of the mandible. They usually lie over the submandibular gland although intracapsular nodes are also possible. The submandibular chain, along with some inconstant small facial nodes, drain the skin and mucous membrane of the nose, medial portion of the eyelid, cheek, upper lip, lateral part of the lower lip,

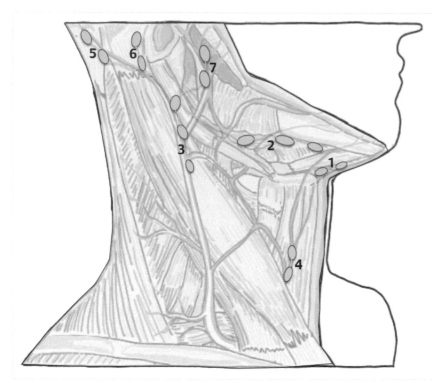

Fig. 2.4 Superficial lymphatics of the neck. 1, submental; 2, submandibular; 3, external jugular; 4, anterior jugular; 5, occipital; 6, mastoid; 7, parotid.

gums, and anterior third of the lateral border of the tongue. These nodes drain into the transverse cervical and deep cervical chains.

The *external jugular nodes* are located between the lower parotid nodes and the midportion of the sternocleidomastoid muscle, along the external jugular vein. They drain the lower part of the ear and the parotid gland into the superior deep cervical chain.

The *anterior jugular nodes* are located on the anteroinferior portion of the neck, parallel to the anterior jugular vein. They drain the infrahyoid area toward the inferior deep jugular chain.

The *occipital nodes* drain the skin of the occipital region and part of the superficial and deep lymphatics of the nape.

The *mastoid nodes* are located over the mastoid process and drain the ear, external auditory canal, and skin of the temporal region.

The *parotid group* includes both superficial and deep nodes. The superficial nodes are located over the external surface of the parotid gland, whereas the deep nodes are intraglandular and accompany the intraparotid course of the retromandibular and external jugular. The parotid nodes drain the skin of the temporal and frontal area, eyelid, auricle, middle ear, parotid, and the mucous surface of the nasal cavity.

Deep Lymphatics

The deep lymphatics drain the mucous membranes of the upper aerodigestive tract, along with organs such as the thyroid and larynx, into the deep cervical lymph node chains. These include the internal jugular, spinal accessory, transverse cervical, retropharyngeal, and deep anterior lymphatic chains (► Fig. 2.5).

The *internal jugular chain* is formed by a variable number of lymph nodes—between 30 and 60—located around the internal jugular vein. The most posterior and smaller nodes are located over the splenius, levator scapulae, and scalene muscles, whereas the anterior nodes are in close relation with the anterior wall of the internal jugular vein. The posterior nodes drain the skin of the back of the head and receive efferent vessels from the occipital and mastoid nodes, as well as cutaneous and muscular tributaries from the neck. The anterior nodes drain the superficial and deep structures of the anterior part of the head and neck, both directly and indirectly.

At the intersection between the digastric muscle and the internal jugular vein there is a constant prominent node, known as the *jugulodigastric* or *Küttner node*. It drains the base of the tongue and the palatine tonsil. Another prominent node, the *juguloomohyoid* or *Poirier node*, is located further down at the crossing of the omohyoid muscle with the internal jugular vein. It receives lymph flow coming from the tongue and submental region.

For practical purposes, the internal jugular chain may be divided into upper, middle, and lower parts, with the dividing lines located at the jugulodigastric and juguloomohyoid nodes. The nodes of the lower part of the internal jugular chain are less constant and participate also in the drainage of noncervical adjacent structures.

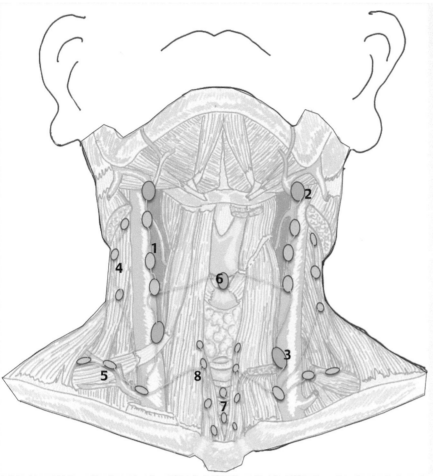

Fig. 2.5 Deep lymphatics of the neck. 1, internal jugular chain; 2, jugulodigastric node; 3, juguloomohyoid node; 4, spinal accessory chain; 5, transverse cervical chain; 6, Delphian node; 7, pretracheal nodes; 8, paratracheal nodes.

The *spinal accessory chain* follows the spinal accessory nerve in the upper part of the posterior triangle and merges with the transverse cervical chain beneath the trapezius muscle. It receives lymph from the occipital and mastoid areas.

The *transverse cervical chain* runs along the transverse cervical vessels. It receives efferent vessels from the spinal accessory chain and from the lateral part of the neck.

The *retropharyngeal nodes* are located at the lateral portion of the parapharyngeal space. They drain the nasal cavity, soft palate, paranasal sinuses, middle ear, nasopharynx, and oropharynx.

The *deep anterior chain* includes the prelaryngeal (Delphian) node, the pretracheal, and the paratracheal nodes. They drain the subglottis, the trachea, and the thyroid gland. This chain is connected with the internal jugular chain.

Major Lymph Ducts

Both, the superficial and the deep lymphatic system initially drain in the nearest lymph nodes and then proceed to more central nodes to finally form lymphatic trunks. At the base of the right side of the neck, the jugular trunk (which collects most of the lymph from one side of the

head and neck), the transverse cervical trunk, and the subclavian trunk frequently join to form the *right lymphatic duct* or *great lymphatic vein*. This large collector courses along the medial border of the scalene muscle and empties into the venous system at the junction of the right internal jugular vein and the right subclavian vein.

The *thoracic duct* begins in the abdomen, passes through the thoracic region, and emerges in the root of the left side of the neck between the common carotid and subclavian arteries. It then arches above the subclavian artery and in front of the vertebral artery and thyrocervical trunk, to pass behind the carotid sheath between the internal jugular vein and the anterior scalene muscle. The thoracic duct empties laterally into the venous system at the junction of the left subclavian and internal jugular veins. The left jugular trunk, left transverse cervical trunk, and left subclavian trunk drain in the thoracic duct or directly in the jugulo-subclavian junction.

2.2.3 Lymph Node Distribution: Nodal Groups

For practical reasons, the neck may be artificially divided into different lymph node regions. This does not mean that there is a true anatomical or physiological separation within the lymphatic system of the neck. On the contrary, a widespread interconnection exists between the different nodal chains, as already described. Thus, the regional lymph node classification should be regarded only as a schematic representation of the lymphatic system of the neck, and not as an anatomical transcription of the reality. As often happens in medicine, nature is much more complex than we would like it to be.

The most popular terminology for subdividing the lymph node groups was proposed by the Memorial Sloan Kettering group in the 1980s, further developed in 1991 by the Committee for Head and Neck Surgery and Oncology of the American Academy of Otolaryngology—Head and Neck Surgery, and reviewed in 2002 and 2008 by a collaboration of the Neck Dissection Committee of the American Head and Neck Society. According to this classification, the neck is divided into six different levels (▶ Fig. 2.6, ▶ Fig. 2.7), three of them additionally subdivided into two sublevels:

- *Sublevel IA: Submental nodes.* This group includes the lymph nodes located within the submental triangle, bounded by the anterior belly of both digastric muscles and by the hyoid bone.
- *Sublevel IB: Submandibular nodes.* The submandibular group includes the lymph nodes located within the boundaries of the anterior and posterior bellies of the digastric muscle, the stylohyoid muscle, and the body of the mandible. These nodes are located around the submandibular gland, which should be removed when this nodal group is included in the resection.

- *Level II: Upper jugular nodes.* This group contains the lymph nodes located around the upper third of the internal jugular vein and the spinal accessory nerve. It goes from the level of the skull base superiorly to the level of the inferior border of the hyoid bone and/or carotid bifurcation inferiorly. The posterior boundary is the posterior border of the sternocleidomastoid muscle, and the anterior boundary is the lateral border of the stylohyoid muscle. This level is divided by the spinal accessory nerve into two sublevels:
  - *Sublevel IIA:* nodes located anterior-medial to the vertical plane defined by the spinal accessory nerve.
  - *Sublevel IIB:* nodes located posterior-lateral to the plane of the nerve.
- *Level III: Middle jugular nodes.* The lymph nodes around the middle third of the internal jugular vein, between the limits of the levels II and IV. The posterior boundary is the posterior border of the sternocleidomastoid muscle and/or the plane defined by the sensory branches of the cervical plexus. The anterior boundary is the lateral border of the sternohyoid muscle and/or the common carotid artery.
- *Level IV: Lower jugular nodes.* This nodal group contains the lymphatic structures located around the lower third of the internal jugular vein. Its upper limit is the inferior border of the cricoid cartilage and/or the point at which the superior belly of the omohyoid muscle crosses the internal jugular vein. The inferior boundary is the clavicle, while the posterior and anterior boundaries are the same as in level III.

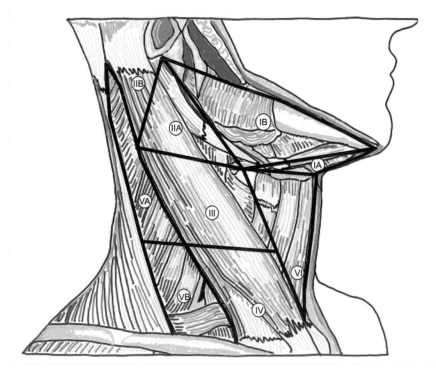

Fig. 2.6 Regional division of the lymphatic system of the neck according to the classification of the American Academy of Otolaryngology—Head and Neck Surgery and the American Head and Neck Society: lateral view. Level IA, submental region; Level IB, submandibular region; Level II, upper jugular region; Level III, middle jugular region; Level IV, lower jugular region; Level V, posterior triangle.

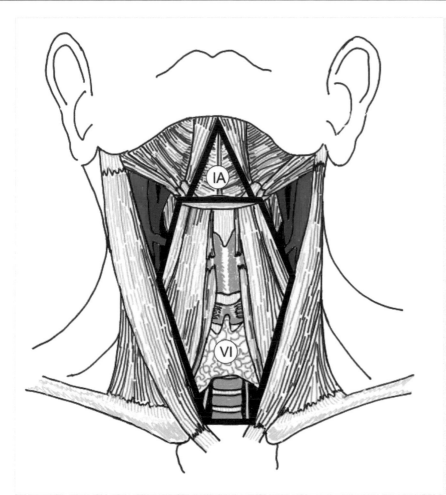

Fig. 2.7 Regional division of the lymphatic system of the neck according to the classification of the American Academy of Otolaryngology—Head and Neck Surgery and the American Head and Neck Society: anterior view. Level IA, submental region; Level VI, central compartment.

- *Level V: Posterior triangle.* The boundaries are the anterior border of the trapezius muscle posteriorly, the posterior border of the sternocleidomastoid muscle and/or the plane of the sensory branches of the cervical plexus anteriorly, and the clavicle inferiorly. This level is subdivided by a horizontal plane at the inferior level of the cricoid cartilage into two sublevels:
  - *Sublevel VA:* includes the lymph nodes located along the lower half of the spinal accessory nerve.
  - *Sublevel VB:* includes the nodes following the transverse cervical vessels, as well as the supraclavicular lymph nodes.
- *Level VI: Anterior or central compartment.* This level contains the prelaryngeal (Delphian) node, and the pre- and paratracheal nodes, including perithyroidal nodes, and the lymph nodes along the recurrent laryngeal nerves. The boundaries are the hyoid bone superiorly, the suprasternal notch inferiorly, and the common carotid arteries laterally.
- *Level VII.* Some authors consider this an additional area. It includes the upper mediastinal lymph nodes located below the suprasternal notch and above the innominate artery.

One of the main theoretical advantages of the nodal group classification is that every group of nodes may be related to different head-and-neck structures in order to assess the potential risk for metastasis for every primary location. ▶ Table 2.1 shows the relationship between the location of the primary tumor and the nodal groups at greatest risk for harboring metastases.

A Final Comment on the Nodal Group Classification

The main use of the nodal group classification is to support the worthiness of selective neck dissections. However, the artificial nature of the division creates some inconsistencies that must be kept in mind to avoid falling into a "nodal group fundamentalism," which often happens nowadays under the name of "super-selective neck dissections." In our opinion, the following are the main weak points of the artificial division of the neck into nodal regions.

1. Despite the effort to correlate surgical and radiological landmarks in the nodal group classification, there is a notorious lack of consistency into this correlation. This

2

Table 2.1 Nodal groups at greatest risk of developing metastases according to the location of the primary tumor

Nodal region	Location of the primary tumor
Area I:	
Submental nodes	Floor of mouth, anterior oral cavity, lower lip
Submandibular nodes	Oral cavity, anterior nasal cavity, mid-face, submandibular gland
Area II: Upper jugular nodes	Oral cavity, nasal cavity, nasopharynx, oropharynx, hypopharynx, larynx, parotid gland
Area III: Middle jugular nodes	Oral cavity, nasopharynx, oropharynx, hypopharynx, larynx
Area IV: Lower jugular nodes	Hypopharynx, larynx, cervical esophagus, thyroid gland
Area V: Posterior triangle	Nasopharynx, oropharynx, skin of posterior scalp and neck
Area VI: Anterior compartment	Thyroid gland, larynx (glottic and subglottic), apex of the piriform sinus, cervical esophagus

makes it very difficult to compare results, even if we all use the same classification. At surgery, the theoretically well-defined anatomical and radiological boundaries of some of the various levels and sublevels are distorted by the operative maneuvers. It is not unusual to decide to stop the dissection at a given point to find later that more tissue than desired has been removed because too much traction has been used during the dissection. On the other hand, even in the ideal situation, one person's upper level IV lymph node may easily be another's lower level III node.

2. Under normal conditions, the lymph flow follows a rather predictable course that is used as an argument to support the oncological safety of selective neck dissections. However, head-and-neck cancer patients do not fully satisfy the criteria of "normal conditions," and the flow pattern may be modified by factors related to the tumor itself, the anatomical characteristics of the patient, and the influence of external factors such as previous treatment. Some operations have stood the test of time and can be considered positively safe from an oncological standpoint. Others still need documented proof of efficacy. Meanwhile, the use of super-selective operations should be cautiously recommended.

3. Finally, the ultimate rationale for selective operations should not be sought on the nodal region subdivision, but on the functional concept. If selective neck dissections are useful—and for some of them this is a fact—it is because the functional concept is a reality. We can remove the lymphatic tissue from the neck without the need to remove adjacent cervical structures. The exact limits of this removal for every single head-and-neck tumor have not been determined with certainty and require further studies and well-designed investigations.

2.3 Anatomical Basis for Functional and Selective Neck Dissection

2.3.1 Topographic Anatomy

The topographic description of the neck intends to serve as a guide in which the external and readily accessible superficial features of the neck provide essential landmarks for deep structures. This is a critical element in the examination and description of clinical findings.

From a topographic standpoint, the sternocleidomastoid muscle and the carotid sheath divide each side of the neck into two different spaces. Although pyramidal in shape, these spaces are known as the anterior and posterior triangles of the neck (▶ Fig. 2.8). The posterior-lateral space has a cranial apex at the level of the mastoid and a base at the level of the clavicle. It does not have a definite anatomical boundary, because it merges into the axilla through the cervicoaxillary canal. The apex of the anterior-medial space is located at the bottom of the neck and its base lies at the level of the submandibular gland and tail of the parotid gland. These spaces contain the lymph nodes that drain most cervical structures.

Anterior Triangle

The anterior triangle is bounded by the anterior midline of the neck, the anterior border of the sternocleidomastoid muscle, and the inferior border of the mandible. The jugular notch constitutes the apex, and the base is formed by the inferior border of the mandible. The posterior belly of the digastric muscle and the superior belly of the omohyoid further divide this space into several smaller triangles (i.e., submental, submandibular, carotid, and muscular; ▶ Fig. 2.9).

The *submental triangle* is an unpaired space bounded on each side by the anterior belly of the digastric muscle, inferiorly by the body of the hyoid bone, and superiorly by the inferior border of the mandible. The floor of the submental triangle is formed by the mylohyoid muscles, which meet in a median fibrous raphe. This space is occupied by fat and lymph nodes.

The *submandibular triangle* is limited on each side by the inferior border of the mandible and the anterior and posterior bellies of the digastric muscle. The muscular floor of the submandibular triangle is formed, from anterior to posterior, by the mylohyoid, hyoglossus, and middle constrictor of the pharynx. The mylohyoid muscle further divides it into supramylohyoid and inframylohyoid spaces. The supramylohyoid space contains the sublingual gland. The submandibular gland and a variable number of lymph nodes are contained within the inframylohyoid space. The lingual nerve, the hypoglossal nerve, part of the facial artery and vein, and the submental artery pass through this triangle.

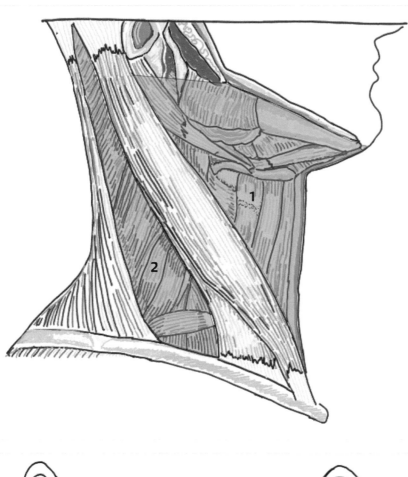

Fig. 2.8 Main topographic division of the neck: 1, anterior triangle; 2, posterior triangle.

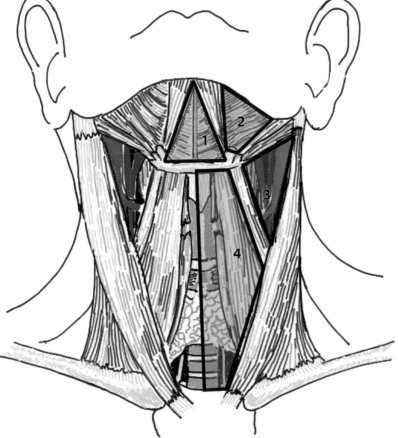

Fig. 2.9 Topographic distribution of the anterior triangle of the neck: 1, submental triangle; 2, submandibular triangle; 3, carotid triangle; 4, muscular triangle.

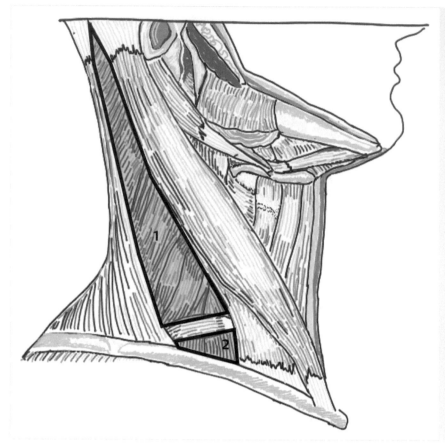

Fig. 2.10 Topographic distribution of the posterior triangle of the neck: 1, occipital triangle; 2, omoclavicular triangle.

The *carotid triangle* (also known as the superior carotid triangle) is bounded superiorly by the posterior belly of the digastric muscle, inferiorly by the superior belly of the omohyoid muscle, and posteriorly by the anterior border of the sternocleidomastoid muscle. The carotid triangle provides an important surgical approach to the carotid system. Many important structures, such as the common carotid artery, internal jugular vein, vagus nerve, and sympathetic trunk, lie within the limits of this space. The common carotid artery divides into the internal and external branches at the level of the superior border of the thyroid cartilage. Many deep cervical lymph nodes lie along the internal jugular vein, and between the vein and the common carotid artery, within the carotid sheath.

The *muscular triangle* (or inferior carotid triangle) is bounded by the superior belly of the omohyoid muscle, the anterior border of the sternocleidomastoid muscle, and the midline of the neck. It contains the strap muscles, the thyroid and parathyroid glands, the larynx and the hypopharynx, the trachea, and the cervical esophagus.

Posterior Triangle

The *posterior cervical triangle* is bounded anteriorly by the posterior border of the sternocleidomastoid muscle, posteriorly by the anterior border of the trapezius, and inferiorly by the middle third of the clavicle. Its floor is formed, from superior to inferior, by the splenius capitis, the

levator scapulae, and the medial and posterior scalene muscles.

The inferior belly of the omohyoid muscle crosses the space, dividing it into two smaller triangles, the occipital triangle above and the omoclavicular or subclavian triangle below (▶ Fig. 2.10). The *occipital triangle* contains the spinal accessory nerve and part of the cervical and brachial plexuses. The occipital artery crosses the upper part of this triangle. The *omoclavicular triangle* corresponds to the supraclavicular fossa.

2.3.2 Surgical Anatomy

This section describes, in the order of appearance, the anatomical structures found by the surgeon in the course of functional and selective neck dissection.

The Skin

The vascular supply of the skin of the neck is provided by descending branches of the facial, submental, and occipital arteries and by ascending branches of the transverse cervical and suprascapular arteries.

The surgeon must take into consideration the blood supply of the skin when planning the incision. Access to the primary tumor and incisions for lymph node dissection should be designed to avoid skin complications. Every effort should be made to design a skin incision that crosses

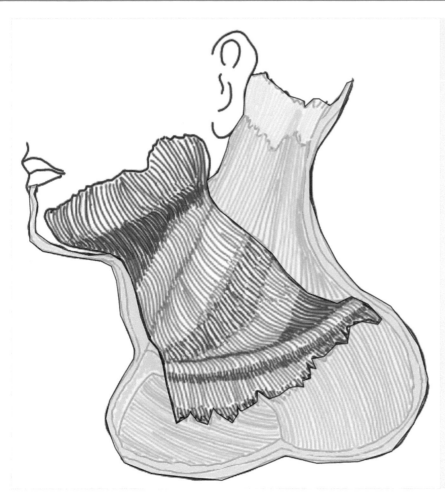

Fig. 2.11 Platysma muscle.

the carotid artery only once on each side, with the crossing point located as far as possible from the carotid artery bifurcation. Whenever possible, incision trifurcations should be avoided.

Platysma Muscle

The *platysma* is a wide, thin sheet of muscle located in the anterolateral aspect of the neck, immediately below the skin and over the superficial layer of the deep cervical fascia (▶ Fig. 2.11). It runs obliquely from the skin and fascia of the pectoralis and deltoid muscle to the lower border of the mandible and skin of the lower face. The platysma muscle is innervated by the cervical branch of the facial nerve.

Raising the skin flap between the platysma muscle and the superficial layer of the deep cervical fascia, on which it rests, allows the identification of the following anatomical structures: external and anterior jugular vein, great auricular nerve, and marginal branch of the facial nerve.

External Jugular Vein

The external jugular vein begins near the angle of the mandible, within the parotid gland, by the junction of the posterior division of the retromandibular vein (posterior facial vein) with the posterior auricular vein (▶ Fig. 2.12). It then runs obliquely across the sternocleidomastoid muscle, within the superficial layer of the deep cervical fascia, parallel and right anteriorly to the great auricular nerve in its upper half. The vein pierces the deep fascial layer at the posterior border of the muscle, about 5 cm above the clavicle. It usually terminates in the subclavian vein, but it may also end in the internal jugular vein. It may be double or have a bifid termination. Sometimes the external jugular vein is very small and may even be absent. In these cases, the anterior jugular vein, the internal jugular vein, or both are usually enlarged. Tributaries and communicating branches to the external jugular vein include the posterior auricular, occipital, posterior external jugular, transverse cervical, suprascapular, and anterior jugular veins.

Anterior Jugular Vein

The anterior jugular vein begins below the chin and communicates with the submental, mental, inferior labial, and hyoid veins (▶ Fig. 2.13). It descends near the midline, within the superficial layer of the deep cervical fascia. Just above the clavicle it turns laterally, piercing the fascial layer, and passing deep to the sternocleidomastoid muscle

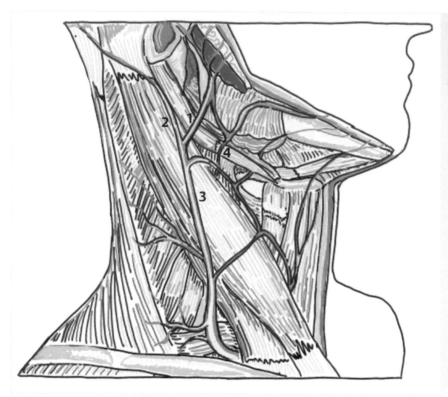

Fig. 2.12 External jugular vein:
1, retromandibular or posterior facial vein;
2, posterior auricular vein; 3, external jugular
vein; 4, facial vein (tributary of the internal
jugular vein).

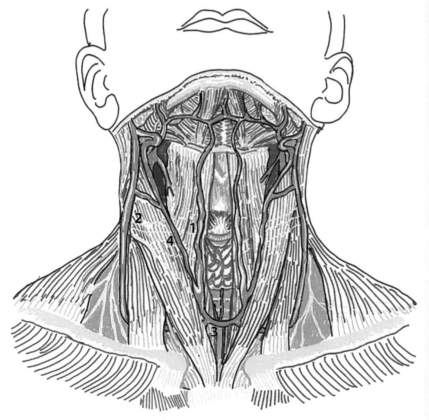

Fig. 2.13 Superficial venous system of the neck:
1, anterior jugular vein; 2, external jugular vein;
3, jugular venous arch; 4, communicating vein
(Kocher vein).

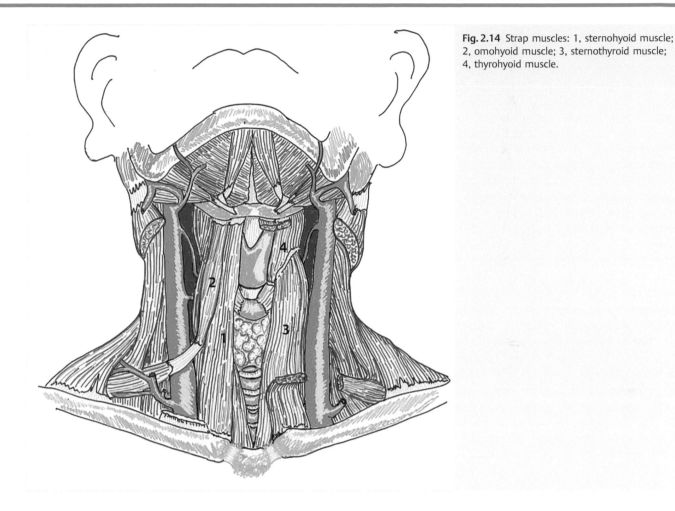

Fig. 2.14 Strap muscles: 1, sternohyoid muscle; 2, omohyoid muscle; 3, sternothyroid muscle; 4, thyrohyoid muscle.

to finally open into the external jugular vein just before its junction with the subclavian vein. As it turns laterally, the anterior jugular vein sends a branch across the midline to join the anterior jugular vein of the opposite side, forming the jugular venous arch.

There is often a connection between the external and anterior jugular veins, known as Kocher vein, which runs through the anterior border of the sternocleidomastoid muscle.

Strap Muscles

The strap muscles (▶ Fig. 2.14), also known as infrahyoid muscles, are enveloped by the middle layer of the deep cervical fascia. Their function is primarily related to the stability of the hyoid bone and larynx during swallowing and speaking. They are innervated by branches of the *ansa cervicalis*.

The *sternohyoid muscle* is the most superficial and medial of the strap muscles. It originates in the body of the hyoid bone and attaches inferiorly to the manubrium of the sternum and medial end of the clavicle.

The *omohyoid muscle* extends between the hyoid bone and the superior margin of the scapula, near the transverse ligament of the scapula. It has two bellies united by an intermediate tendon. The superior belly of the omohyoid descends posterolateral to the sternohyoid muscle, parallel to it and covering the thyrohyoid and sternothyroid muscles. The intermediate tendon is located beneath the sternocleidomastoid muscle and crosses superficial to the internal jugular vein. This tendon is held in place by a strong reinforcement of the middle layer of the cervical fascia, which binds it to the posterior surface of the clavicle. The inferior belly of the omohyoid muscle crosses the brachial plexus and the scalene muscles, and is partly covered by the trapezius in its distal end.

The *sternothyroid muscle* takes its origin from the dorsal surface of the manubrium and inserts by short tendinous fibers into the oblique line on the lamina of the thyroid cartilage. It lies superficial to the brachiocephalic vein, the trachea, and the thyroid gland.

The *thyrohyoid muscle* continues the sternothyroid muscle superiorly. It is largely covered by the omohyoid and sternohyoid muscles. It takes its origin from the oblique line on the lamina of the thyroid cartilage and inserts into the inferior margin of the lateral third of the body of the hyoid bone.

Cervical Plexus: Superficial Branches

The cervical plexus is a neural network formed by the communications between the ventral rami of the superior four cervical nerves, which form loops with one another. It has both deep and superficial branches. The deep motor branches are the ansa cervicalis and the phrenic nerve, and will be discussed later in this chapter.

The superficial cutaneous branches of the cervical plexus emerge around the midportion of the posterior border of the sternocleidomastoid muscle (Erb's point) to supply the skin of the neck and inferior part of the scalp and the face (▶ Fig. 2.15). These superficial branches diverge into ascending, descending, and transverse ramifications.

The ascending branches include the lesser occipital nerve (C1, C2) and the great auricular nerve (C2, C3). The *lesser occipital nerve* ascends along the posterior margin of the sternocleidomastoid muscle to the mastoid process. It divides into auricular, mastoid, and occipital terminal branches, to provide sensory innervation to these areas. The *great auricular nerve* crosses the superficial surface of the sternocleidomastoid muscle and divides into anterior and posterior branches at the level of the anterior border of the muscle. The posterior branch innervates the mastoid and the posterior surface of the auricle, while the anterior branch goes toward the angle of the mandible to supply the anterior surface of the auricle and the skin of the cheek.

The *transverse cervical nerve* (C2, C3) passes transversely across the sternocleidomastoid muscle and divides into superior and inferior terminal twigs for the skin of the neck.

The *supraclavicular nerve* (C3, C4) constitutes the main descending branch of the cervical plexus. It arises as a single trunk and divides into medial, intermediate, and lateral branches, supplying the skin over the anterior aspect of the chest and shoulder. The medial and lateral supraclavicular nerves also supply the sternoclavicular and acromioclavicular joints, respectively.

Sternocleidomastoid Muscle

The sternocleidomastoid muscle is a broad straplike muscle enveloped by the superficial layer of the deep fascia. The sternocleidomastoid muscle is a key reference in neck surgery. It runs superolaterally from the sternum and clavicle to skull (▶ Fig. 2.16), covering the great vessels of the neck and the deep branches of the cervical plexus. The superior end attaches to the lateral surface of the mastoid process, the temporal bone, and the lateral half of the superior nuchal line of the occipital bone. The inferior end has two different heads. The sternal head attaches to the anterior surface of the manubrium of the sternum, lateral

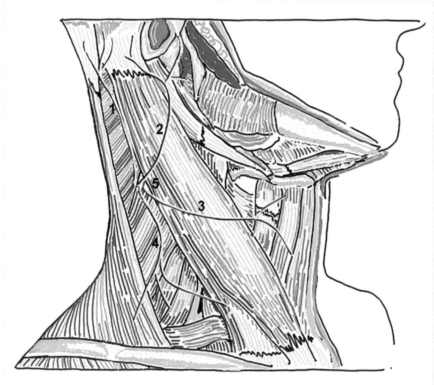

Fig. 2.15 Superficial branches of the cervical plexus: 1, lesser occipital nerve; 2, great auricular nerve; 3, transverse cervical nerve; 4, supraclavicular nerve; 5, Erb's point.

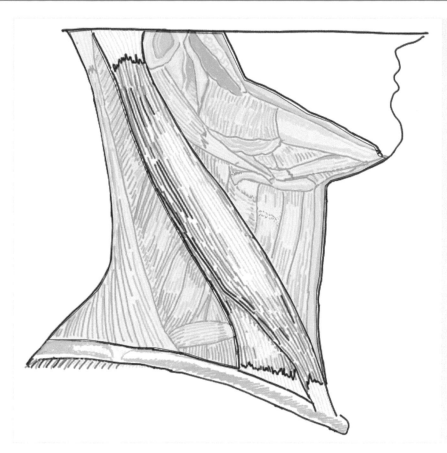

Fig. 2.16 Sternocleidomastoid muscle.

to the jugular notch. The clavicular head attaches to the superior surface of the medial third of the clavicle. The sternocleidomastoid muscle is innervated by the spinal accessory nerve and branches of the second and third cervical nerves.

Submandibular Triangle

The submandibular triangle is located at the upper boundary of the surgical field, with the submandibular gland almost entirely filling its space. The floor of this triangle is formed by the suprahyoid muscles. The hypoglossal and lingual nerves, as well as the lingual vessels, traverse the submandibular triangle and must be identified at surgery. The marginal mandibular branch of the facial nerve lies in the surface of this triangle.

Submandibular Gland

The submandibular gland has a superficial part and a small deep lobe. The superficial portion is variable in size and may be palpated through the skin of the submandibular triangle by applying pressure from the floor of the mouth. The deep lobe is located internal to the mylohyoid muscle.

The lateral surface of the gland is crossed by the facial vein and the marginal mandibular branch of the facial

nerve (▶ Fig. 2.17). The upper lateral surface of the gland is in contact with the submandibular fovea of the medial surface of the mandible and with the caudal part of the medial pterygoid muscle. The dorsal part of the gland is deeply grooved by the facial artery, and it is separated from the parotid gland by the stylomandibular ligament. The deep surface of the submandibular gland is in contact anteriorly with the superficial surface of the mylohyoid muscle, and posteriorly with the hyoglossus, stylohyoid, and posterior belly of the digastric muscle. The mylohyoid nerve and artery as well as the submental artery lie between the gland and the mylohyoid muscle. The hypoglossal nerve, the lingual vein, and the first part of the lingual artery are closely related to the posterior deep surface of the submandibular gland.

The deep lobe of the gland is a tonguelike extension that passes around the posterior border of the mylohyoid muscle and extends anteriorly along with the submandibular duct (▶ Fig. 2.18). This glandular prolongation is located between the mylohyoid muscle (laterally) and the hyoglossus and genioglossus muscles (medially). At first, the deep process lies just caudal to the lingual nerve and submandibular ganglion, and it often extends as far as the sublingual gland.

Inferior and posterior to the submandibular region, the superficial layer of the deep cervical fascia fuses with the fascia of the posterior belly of the digastric and stylohyoid

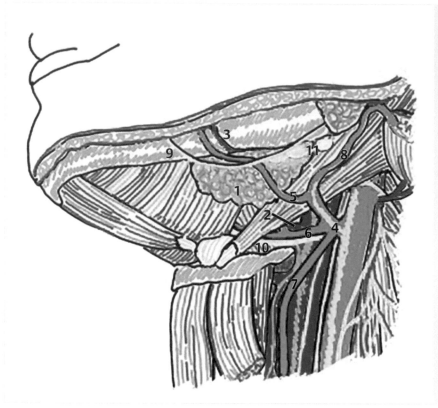

Fig. 2.17 Contents and boundaries of the submandibular triangle of the neck.
1, submandibular gland; 2, lingual artery; 3, facial artery; 4, thyrolinguofacial trunk; 5, facial vein; 6, lingual vein; 7, superior thyroid vein; 8, retromandibular vein; 9, marginal mandibular branch of the facial nerve; 10, hypoglossal nerve; 11, periglandular lymph nodes.

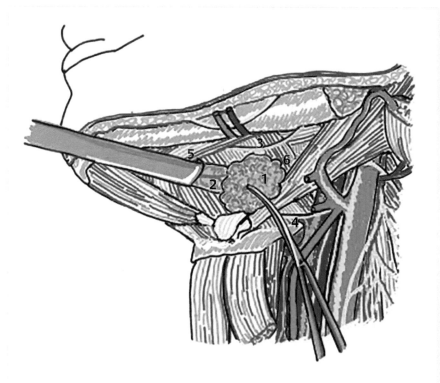

Fig. 2.18 Submandibular triangle after retracting the superficial lobe of the submandibular gland posteriorly, and the mylohyoid muscle anteriorly.
1, superficial lobe of the submandibular gland; 2, deep lobe of the submandibular gland and Wharton duct; 3, lingual nerve; 4, hypoglossal nerve; 5, mylohyoid muscle (retracted); 6, hyoglossus muscle.

muscles and attaches to the hyoid bone. As it bridges the submandibular triangle and passes to the mandible, it splits into two laminae to enclose the submandibular gland, forming its capsule. These laminae attach to the mandible at the margins of the submandibular fovea. Posteriorly, the submandibular space is adjacent to that of the parotid gland, the fascial thickening between them being the stylomandibular ligament. Lymph nodes can be found inside the submandibular cell, on and around the gland (▶ Fig. 2.17). The gland should be included in the resection if these nodes are to be removed. Their involvement by metastatic cancer depends on the location of the primary tumor. As a general rule, the submandibular triangle should be included in the dissection when the primary lesion is located on the anterior portion of the tongue, the floor of the mouth, the lower lip, the tonsil, and the lower anterior portion of the gingiva.

Muscles

Mylohyoid muscle (▶ Fig. 2.19): This flat triangular muscle originates from the mylohyoid ridge of the mandible and inserts into a median raphe and the body of the hyoid bone. It fans out from the anterior surface of the hyoid bone to the posterior aspect of the inferior margin of the mandible. It is covered partially by the submandibular gland, anterior belly of the digastric muscle, and superficial layer of the deep cervical fascia. The submental artery crosses the muscle. It is innervated by the mylohyoid nerve, a branch of the inferior alveolar nerve. The mylohyoid muscle elevates the hyoid bone,

the floor of the mouth, and the tongue during swallowing and speaking.

Hyoglossus muscle (▶ Fig. 2.19): This is a flat quadrangular muscle that forms the posterior floor of the submandibular triangle. It arises from the greater horn of the hyoid bone and runs toward the lateral surface of the tongue, in a direction perpendicular to the mylohyoid muscle and entering deep to it. As a part of the lingual muscles, it is innervated by the hypoglossal nerve.

Geniohyoid muscle: This short and narrow muscle is located superior to the mylohyoid, and it is occult by the latter during neck dissection. It has its origin at the mental spine of the mandible and inserts into the anterior surface of the body of the hyoid bone, where it contacts with the contralateral muscle. It is innervated by the first cervical nerve and pulls the hyoid anterosuperiorly, shortening the floor of the mouth and widening the pharynx.

Digastric muscle (▶ Fig. 2.19): This muscle has two bellies united by an intermediate tendon, which is connected to the body and greater horn of the hyoid bone by a strong loop of fibrous connective tissue. The posterior belly arises by a tendinous process from the mastoid notch of the temporal bone. The fiber bundles form a ribbonlike belly that converges on the intermediate tendon a short distance above the hyoid bone. The posterior belly lies medial to the mastoid and sternocleidomastoid muscle, and lateral to the internal jugular vein, internal carotid artery, and the last three cranial nerves. It is innervated by a branch of the facial nerve given off at the stylomastoid foramen. The intermediate tendon lies deep to the superficial lobe of the submandibular gland and superficial to the hyoglossus and

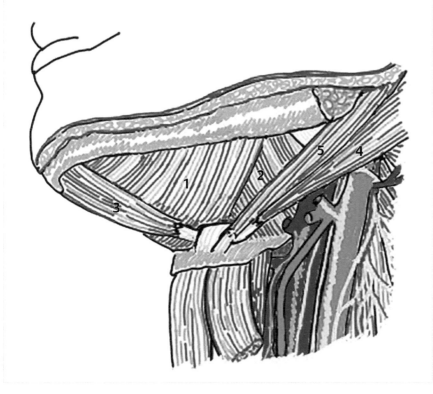

Fig. 2.19 Muscles of the submandibular triangle.
1, mylohyoid muscle; 2, hyoglossus muscle;
3, anterior belly of the digastric muscle;
4, posterior belly of the digastric muscle;
5, stylohyoid muscle.

2

mylohyoid muscles. The anterior belly arises by a short tendinous process from the digastric fossa at the mandible. The fibers converge on both surfaces of the flattened anterior end of the intermediate tendon. The anterior belly lies on the mylohyoid muscle and is covered by the superficial fascia and the platysma muscle. It is innervated by a branch of the mandibular nerve.

Stylohyoid muscle (▶ Fig. 2.19): This muscle takes its origin from the styloid process of the temporal bone, parallels the posterior belly of the digastric muscle, and divides into two slips, which pass on either side of the digastric tendon to attach to the body of the hyoid. It is innervated by a branch of the facial nerve leaving the main trunk as it emerges from the stylomastoid foramen. The stylohyoid muscle elevates and retracts the hyoid bone, elongating the floor of the mouth.

Nerves

The *marginal mandibular branch of the facial nerve* is a thin nerve that provides motion to the lower lip and chin. A precise knowledge of its location is crucial during functional neck dissection because it runs parallel to the superior border of the surgical field. The nerve crosses the surface of the submandibular triangle in its superior part, parallel to the inferior border of the body of the mandible. It courses deep to the superficial layer of the cervical fascia, but superficial to the adventitia of the anterior facial vein (▶ Fig. 2.17). This is an important key to help preservation of the nerve at surgery.

The *hypoglossal nerve* crosses the submandibular triangle to provide motor innervation for all the muscles of the tongue except the palatoglossus. After leaving the cranial cavity through the hypoglossal canal, the trunk of the nerve emerges between the internal carotid artery and the internal jugular vein. The hypoglossal nerve turns anteriorly and crosses superficial to the vagus nerve and the external carotid artery, immediately inferior to the origin of the occipital artery. The nerve enters the submandibular triangle deep to the posterior belly of the digastric muscle and disappears between the hyoglossus and mylohyoid muscles on its way to the tongue (▶ Fig. 2.17, ▶ Fig. 2.18). Before reaching the muscles of the tongue, the nerve is usually crossed by one or more lingual veins that may be a source of troublesome bleeding at surgery.

The *lingual nerve* is the smallest terminal branch of the posterior division of the V3. It provides general sensory fibers to the anterior two-thirds of the tongue, the floor of the mouth, and the gingiva of the mandibular teeth. At first it descends on the medial side of the lateral pterygoid muscle, to pass between the medial pterygoid muscle and the ramus of the mandible toward the posterior part of the mylohyoid line. At this point it is situated a short distance posterior to the last molar tooth and is covered by the mucous membrane of the oral cavity. After leaving the

medial pterygoid muscle, it crosses the lateral superior constrictor muscle of the pharynx and turns toward the tip of the tongue, crossing the lateral surface of the styloglossus, hyoglossus, and genioglossus muscles. As it crosses the hyoglossus muscle, it first lies superior to, then to the lateral side of, and finally inferior to the duct of the submandibular gland. As it ascends on the genioglossus muscle, it lies on the medial side of the duct. This nerve can be found in the submandibular triangle after retracting posteriorly the submandibular gland and anteriorly the mylohyoid muscle (▶ Fig. 2.18); the lingual nerve is attached to the submandibular gland by small branches from the nerve to the submandibular ganglion and from here to the gland. These latter branches carry parasympathetic fibers that reach the lingual nerve through the chorda tympani and innervate the submandibular gland.

Vessels

The *lingual artery* (▶ Fig. 2.17) is the second branch of the external carotid artery, arising at the level of the greater horn of the hyoid bone, below or covered by the posterior belly of the digastric muscle and the angle of the mandible. From here it runs forward or curves upward, giving off branches to the base of the tongue. It enters the tongue above the hyoid bone, deep to the hyoglossus muscle and hypoglossal nerve. At the tip of the tongue the terminal part of the lingual artery, called the deep lingual artery, forms an anastomotic loop with the contralateral artery. The sublingual artery arises from the lingual artery at the anterior border of the hyoglossus muscle. It runs anterosuperiorly to supply the sublingual gland and the adjacent muscles.

The *lingual vein* begins near the tip of the tongue, where it accompanies the deep lingual artery. It first lies beneath the mucous membrane covering the lower surface of the tongue. Then, it courses with the lingual artery deep to the hyoglossus muscle. In the vicinity of the posterior border of this muscle, it receives the dorsal lingual veins coming from the dorsum of the tongue, pharyngeal wall, and palatine tonsils. At the posterior border of the hyoglossus muscle, the lingual vein is joined by the accompanying veins of the hypoglossal nerve. The lingual vein flows into the internal jugular vein, usually by means of a common trunk with the facial and superior thyroid veins (▶ Fig. 2.17).

Spinal Accessory Nerve

The eleventh cranial nerve is called the spinal accessory nerve because of if its dual origin, for it has a cranial root and a spinal root. It is exclusively motor. The spinal or inferior root emerges from the lateral aspect of the spinal cord dorsal to the denticulate ligament. As the fibers emerge, they unite to form an ascending strand, which enters the posterior cranial fossa through the foramen magnum. The strand turns laterally and unites with the cranial part (coming from the nucleus ambiguus) to exit the cranial cavity through the jugular foramen.

After crossing the jugular foramen, the eleventh cranial nerve immediately divides into two branches. The internal branch, which contains the fibers of the cranial root, joins the vagus nerve, and the fibers are distributed to the larynx through the recurrent laryngeal nerve. The external branch, which contains the fibers of the spinal root, innervates the sternocleidomastoid and the trapezius muscles.

The *external branch of the spinal accessory nerve* is the one that can be found during neck dissection. From the jugular foramen, it runs dorsally and laterally, crossing the internal jugular vein at a point covered by the posterior belly of the digastric muscle and superficial to the transverse process of the atlas (▶ Fig. 2.20). The nerve has been found to cross anterior to the jugular vein in approximately two-thirds of the cases,

posterior to the vein in a quarter of the patients, or even piercing the vein in less than 5% of the situations (▶ Fig. 2.21). While it crosses to the lateral side of the internal jugular vein, it may pass anterior or posterior to the occipital artery.

After crossing the internal jugular vein, the accessory nerve descends obliquely downward and backward to the upper part of the sternocleidomastoid muscle. It gives off a branch into the deep surface of this muscle and passes downward and backward, either deep to the sternocleidomastoid or through it, to course across the posterior triangle. The nerve leaves the sternocleidomastoid muscle above Erb's point, where the superficial branches of the cervical plexus turn around the posterior border of the muscle (▶ Fig. 2.22). In the posterior triangle the nerve runs a superficial course reaching the anterior border of the trapezius 2 cm above the clavicle.

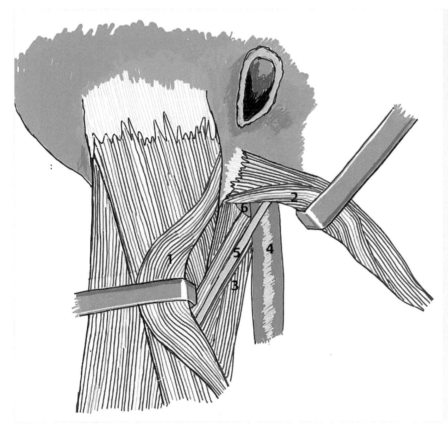

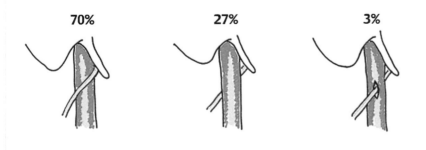

70% **27%** **3%**

Fig. 2.20 External branch of the spinal accessory nerve between the jugular foramen and the sternocleidomastoid muscle.
1, sternocleidomastoid muscle (retracted laterally); 2, posterior belly of digastric muscle (retracted superiorly); 3, splenius capitis muscle; 4, internal jugular vein; 5, spinal accessory nerve; 6, transverse process of the atlas.

Fig. 2.21 Anatomic relations between the spinal accessory nerve and the internal jugular vein.

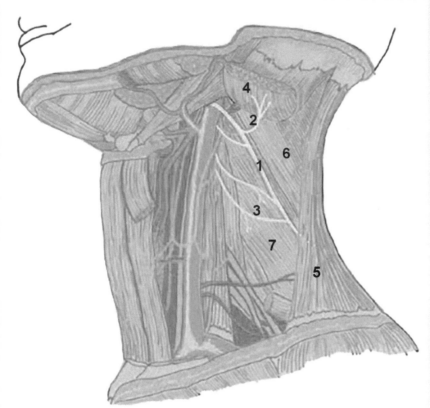

Fig. 2.22 Course of the spinal accessory nerve in the posterior triangle. 1, spinal accessory nerve; 2, branch to the sternocleidomastoid muscle; 3, deep branches of the cervical plexus anastomosing with the spinal accessory nerve; 4, sternocleidomastoid muscle (severed); 5, trapezius muscle; 6, splenius capitis muscle; 7, levator scapulae muscle.

Posterior Triangle of the Neck

The posterior triangle of the neck is bounded by the sternocleidomastoid muscle, the anterior border of the trapezius, and the middle third of the clavicle (▶ Fig. 2.23).

The deep muscular floor of the posterior triangle is formed (superior to inferior) by the splenius capitis, the levator scapulae muscle, and the scalene muscles, covered by the prevertebral part of the deep cervical fascia (▶ Fig. 2.24).

The *splenius capitis* muscle forms the upper portion of the floor of the posterior triangle. It has its origin in the inferior half of the ligamentum nuchae and spinous processes of the upper six thoracic vertebrae and goes to the lateral aspect of the mastoid and lateral third of the superior nuchal line. It is innervated by dorsal rami of the inferior cervical nerves.

The *levator scapulae* muscle arises from the posterior tubercles of the transverse processes of C1 to C4, and goes to the superior part of the medial border of the scapula. It runs medial and inferior to the splenius capitis. Between both muscles there is a "step" that may be identified during the dissection of the posterior triangle of the neck. The levator scapulae muscle is innervated by the dorsal scapular (C5) and cervical spinal (C3 and C4) nerves.

The *scalene muscles* constitute a triangular block that extends between the first two ribs and the transverse processes of the cervical vertebrae, and forms most of the floor of the posterior triangle. The scalene group is formed by three different muscles: the anterior, medial, and posterior scalene muscles.

The *anterior scalene* muscle arises from the anterior tubercles of the transverse processes of the fourth, fifth, and sixth cervical vertebrae and inserts into the scalene tubercle on the upper surface of the body of the first rib.

The *middle scalene* muscle arises from the lateral edge of the costotransverse lamellae of the lower five cervical vertebrae and, like the anterior scalene, goes to the upper surface of the first rib behind the subclavian groove. The lower insertion usually extends to the second rib. It is innervated by the ventral rami of the fourth, fifth, sixth, seventh, and eighth cervical nerves and lies posterior to the ventral roots of the brachial plexus and the third part of the subclavian artery.

The *posterior scalene* muscle is the smallest and deepest of the three scalene muscles. It arises by short tendons from the posterior tubercles of the transverse processes of the fifth and sixth cervical vertebrae but may have its origin as high as the fourth vertebra or as low as the seventh. It is inserted by a short tendon into the lateral surface of the second rib or, occasionally, into the third rib.

The spinal accessory nerve, the internal jugular vein, and the occipital artery are the most important anatomical landmarks in the upper part of the posterior triangle. The deep branches of the cervical plexus run over the muscular floor of the posterior triangle, deep to the internal jugular vein and sternocleidomastoid muscle.

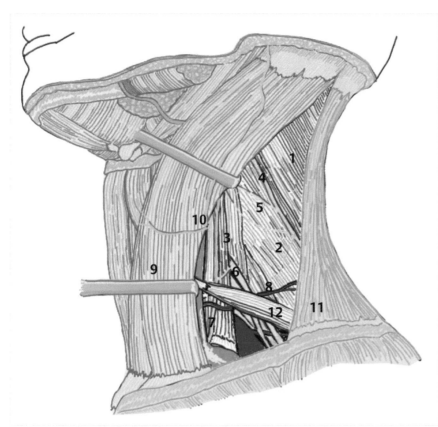

Fig. 2.23 Contents and boundaries of the posterior triangle of the neck. 1, splenius capitis muscle; 2, levator scapulae muscle; 3, scalene muscles; 4, spinal accessory nerve; 5, deep branches of the cervical plexus; 6, brachial plexus; 7, phrenic nerve; 8, transverse cervical artery; 9, sternocleidomastoid muscle; 10, Erb's point; 11, trapezius muscle; 12, inferior belly of the omohyoid muscle.

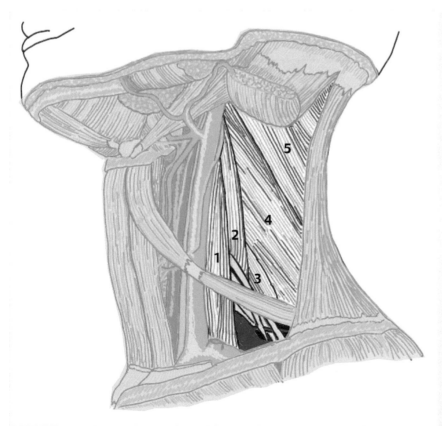

Fig. 2.24 Deep muscles of the neck: 1, anterior scalene muscle; 2, middle scalene muscle; 3, posterior scalene muscle; 4, levator scapulae muscle; 5, splenius capitis muscle.

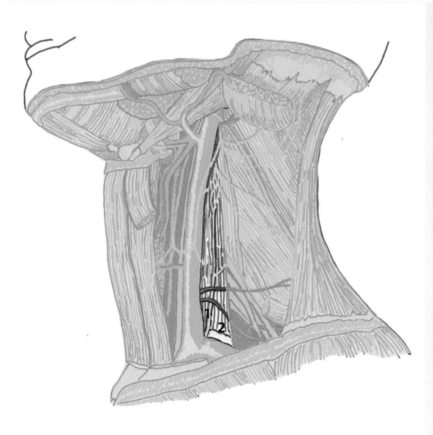

Fig. 2.25 Phrenic nerve as it crosses the neck: 1, phrenic nerve; 2, anterior scalene muscle.

Phrenic Nerve

The phrenic nerve is an important muscular—deep—branch of the cervical plexus (▶ Fig. 2.25) and constitutes the sole motor nerve supply to the diaphragm. It arises mainly from the ventral primary rami of C4, but it has some fibers from C3 and C5. The nerve curves around the lateral border of the anterior scalene muscle and descends obliquely across the anterior surface of the muscle, deep to the transverse cervical and supraclavicular arteries. The phrenic nerve is covered by the deep layer of the cervical fascia. At the root of the neck the phrenic nerve passes off the anterior border of the anterior scalene muscle and descends anterior to the first part of the subclavian artery and the pleura immediately below that artery.

Brachial Plexus

The brachial plexus is formed by the ventral primary rami of C5 to T1 and provides neural supply to the upper limb. The brachial plexus emerges into the posterior triangle between the anterior and middle scalene muscles, and crosses the inferior part of the triangle in an oblique inferior-lateral direction (▶ Fig. 2.23, ▶ Fig. 2.26), covered by the deep cervical fascia. The nerve branches of the brachial plexus are crossed by the lower part of the external jugular vein, the nerve to the subclavius muscle, the transverse cervical vein, the suprascapular vein, the posterior belly of the omohyoid muscle, and the transverse cervical artery. At the root of the neck, the brachial plexus lies posterior to the clavicle, whereas the subclavius muscle and the suprascapular artery cross anterior to the plexus.

Ansa Cervicalis

The ansa cervicalis is part of the cervical plexus (▶ Fig. 2.27). It innervates the strap muscles. The ansa is formed by the union of the descendens hypoglossi, also known as superior ramus of the cervical loop, and the inferior ramus of the cervical loop.

The *superior ramus* of the cervical loop is formed by the union of the ventral rami of the first and second cervical nerves. This nerve travels for some time in the sheath of the hypoglossal nerve. This is the reason why it was called the descendens hypoglossi, but none of the fibers are derived from the hypoglossal nucleus. It arises as the hypoglossal nerve crosses the internal carotid artery and runs inferiorly to join the inferior ramus of the cervical loop.

The *inferior ramus* comes from the loop of the ventral rami of the second and third cranial nerves. The superior and inferior rami interlace to form the *ansa cervicalis*. The

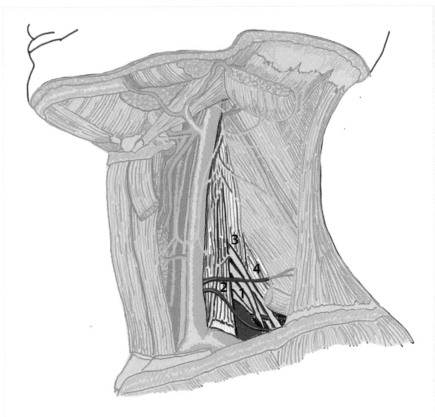

Fig. 2.26 Brachial plexus: 1, brachial plexus; 2, anterior scalene muscle; 3, middle scalene muscle; 4, posterior scalene muscle.

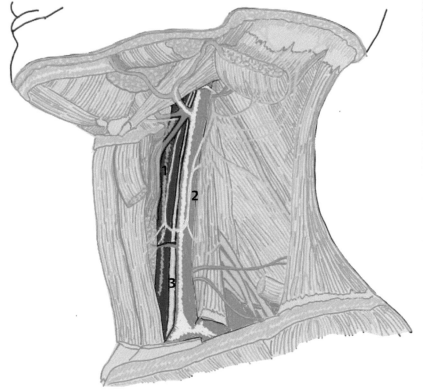

Fig. 2.27 Ansa cervicalis and vagus nerve: 1, superior ramus; 2, inferior ramus; 3, vagus nerve.

2

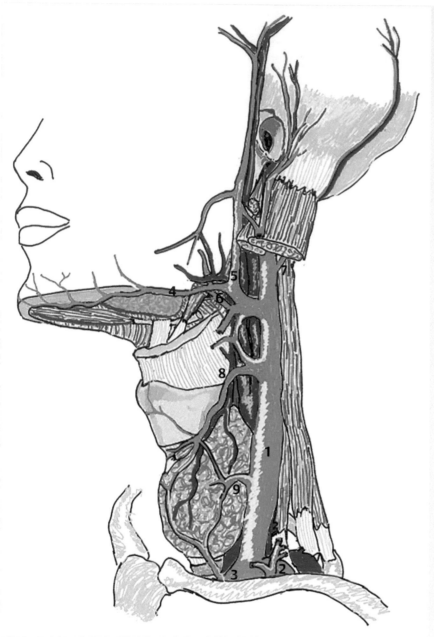

Fig. 2.28 Internal jugular vein and its branches:
1, internal jugular vein; 2, subclavian vein;
3, brachiocephalic trunk; 4, facial vein;
5, retromandibular vein; 6, lingual vein;
7, sternocleidomastoid vein; 8, superior thyroid
vein; 9, middle thyroid vein.

ansa cervicalis may be found between the sternocleido-mastoid muscle and the common carotid artery, superficial to the internal jugular vein.

Carotid Sheath

The structures surrounded by the carotid sheath constitute important anatomical landmarks for functional and selective neck dissection. Precise knowledge of the anatomy of the internal jugular vein, carotid artery and its branches, and vagus nerve is crucial for a successful surgery. The sympathetic trunk, which is closely related to the carotid sheath, may also appear in the surgical field.

Internal Jugular Vein

The internal jugular vein is usually the largest vein in the neck and drains the brain and the superficial parts of the face and neck (▶ Fig. 2.28). It begins at the jugular fossa as the continuation of the sigmoid sinus. The internal jugular vein on the right side of the neck is usually larger because of the greater volume of blood entering from the superior sagittal sinus through the sigmoid sinus.

At first, the internal jugular vein lies in front of the rectus capitis muscle and posterolateral to the internal carotid artery, from which it is separated by the carotid plexus of the sympathetic trunk as well as by the hypoglossal, glossopharyngeal, and vagus nerves. As it descends, it passes gradually to the lateral side of the internal carotid artery first, and to the common carotid artery later, in the same sheath as the artery and vagus nerve, but separated from these structures by a distinct septum. On its way to the base of the neck, the vein gradually overlaps the artery anteriorly.

At the upper part, the internal jugular vein receives the inferior petrosal sinus and a meningeal vein. At the level of the angle of the mandible, it receives some veins from the pharyngeal plexus as well as a communicating branch from the external jugular vein. The facial vein enters the internal jugular vein at the level of the carotid bifurcation. Further inferiorly, the lingual, sternocleidomastoid, and superior thyroid veins join the main trunk of the internal jugular vein. Sometimes these veins enter the internal jugular vein through a common trunk, the thyrolinguofacial trunk, which crosses over the hypoglossal nerve. Along the lateral surface of the thyroid gland, the internal jugular vein is joined by the middle thyroid vein.

The upper portion of the internal jugular vein is covered by the digastric muscle. At the lower part of the neck, the vein is crossed by the omohyoid muscle. The internal jugular vein courses inferiorly through the neck along with the carotid artery, toward the inferior border of the sternoclavicular articulation, where it joins the subclavian vein to form the brachiocephalic trunk.

A large number of lymph nodes lie along the internal jugular vein, in the interstices of the fascial septa of the carotid sheath (▶ Fig. 2.5). Thus, careful dissection of this structure is one of the characteristic surgical steps of functional and selective neck dissection. Longitudinal incision of the carotid sheath allows the removal of the lymph nodes located along the vascular axis of the neck as well as preservation of the important neurovascular structures surrounded by this fascial sheath.

Carotid Artery

The right *common carotid artery* arises at the bifurcation of the brachiocephalic trunk, whereas the left common carotid artery comes from the aortic arch. The common carotid artery has no branches until its termination, keeping the same diameter throughout its full course (▶ Fig. 2.29). The cranial portion of the common carotid artery has a dilatation, known as the carotid sinus, which is characterized by more elastic walls and a special innervation through the carotid sinus branch of the glossopharyngeal nerve. The carotid sinus collaborates in the regulation of blood pressure. The common carotid artery lies medial and posterior to the internal jugular vein at the level of the sternoclavicular joint, running more anterior and medial as it ascends. The vagus nerve is located between the internal jugular vein and the common carotid artery. The common carotid artery ascends in the vascular sheath up to the level of the superior horn of the thyroid

cartilage, where it divides into internal and external branches. After its division, the internal and external carotid arteries ascend in the neck, diverging from each other in a V form and running in an anterior posterior direction.

The *internal carotid artery* is the continuation of the common carotid artery. It has no branches in the neck, and ascends medial and posterior to the internal jugular vein toward the skull base (▶ Fig. 2.29). At its origin it runs lateral and posterior to the external carotid artery, lying on the longus capitis muscle. As it ascends, it passes internal and posterior to the external branch. The internal carotid artery enters the middle cranial fossa through the carotid canal in the petrous portion of the temporal bone.

The *external carotid artery* arises from the carotid sinus at the level of the fourth cervical vertebra. It runs vertical from the superior horn of the thyroid cartilage to the anterior border of the tragus, anterior and medial to the internal carotid artery. It is crossed by the hypoglossal nerve and passes deep to the posterior belly of the digastric and stylohyoid muscles. It is separated from the internal carotid artery by the stylopharyngeus and styloglossus muscles, styloid process, glosso-pharyngeal nerve, and pharyngeal branches of the vagus nerve. The superior laryngeal nerve lies medial to the artery in the carotid triangle. On its final portion the external carotid artery ascends posterior to the angle of the mandible and deep to the parotid gland, diverging laterally to become more superficial. It then perforates the parotid gland and accompanies the retromandibular vein through the gland toward the neck of the mandible, where it terminates by dividing into the superficial temporal and maxillary arteries (▶ Fig. 2.29). Most of the branches of the external carotid artery arise in the carotid triangle. The branches of the external carotid artery in the neck are the superior thyroid, ascending pharyngeal, lingual, occipital, facial, and posterior auricular arteries.

The *superior thyroid artery* arises from the anterior border of the external carotid artery, just inferior to the great horn of the hyoid bone. The artery arches anteriorly and then descends obliquely toward the superior pole of the thyroid gland, deep to the strap muscles. The main branches of the superior thyroid artery are the infrahyoid, sternocleidomastoid, superior laryngeal, cricothyroid, and glandular arteries. The *infrahyoid artery* runs inferior to the hyoid bone lying on the thyrohyoid membrane. The *sternocleidomastoid artery* runs posteriorly to enter the deep surface of the muscle. The *superior laryngeal artery* arises from the arching part of the superior thyroid artery. It passes forward toward the posterior border of the thyrohyoid muscle, along with the superior laryngeal vein and the internal branch of the superior laryngeal nerve. The neurovascular bundle pierces the thyrohyoid membrane and supplies the laryngeal muscles, the inferior pharyngeal constrictor muscle, and the endolaryngeal mucosa. The *cricothyroid artery* runs medially, supplying the cricothyroid muscle and membrane. It crosses the midline

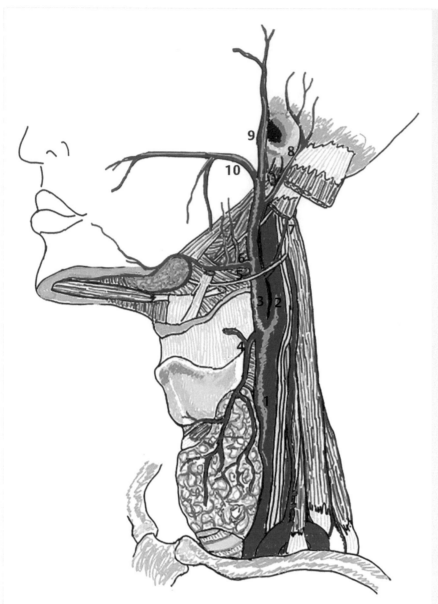

Fig. 2.29 Carotid artery and its branches: 1, common carotid artery; 2, internal carotid artery; 3, external carotid artery; 4, superior thyroid artery; 5, lingual artery; 6, facial artery; 7, occipital artery; 8, posterior auricular artery; 9, superficial temporal artery; 10, maxillary artery.

creating an extralaryngeal anastomotic arch with the branches from the opposite side. The *glandular arteries* are the direct continuation of the superior thyroid artery and constitute the final and largest branches of the superior thyroid artery. They divide at the superior pole of the thyroid gland into anterior and posterior branches.

The *ascending pharyngeal artery* is usually the second branch of the external carotid artery. It is a long, small vessel that arises from the posterior wall of the artery and runs on the pharynx, deep to the internal carotid artery, sending branches to the pharynx, prevertebral muscles, middle ear, and meninges.

The *lingual artery* arises from the anterior wall of the external carotid artery at the level of the greater horn of the hyoid bone, between the superior thyroid and facial arteries. In its first portion it lies on the middle constrictor muscle, covered only by the superficial layer of the deep

cervical fascia and the platysma muscle. It then arches upward, passing deep to the hypoglossal nerve, stylohyoid muscle, and posterior belly of the digastric muscle, to disappear into the depth of the hyoglossus muscle.

The *facial artery* arises from the anterior border of the external carotid artery, just above the lingual artery and sometimes from a common trunk. In the neck, the facial artery lies on the middle and superior constrictor muscles, deep to the stylohyoid and posterior belly of the digastric muscles. It enters the submandibular triangle deep to the posterior part of the submandibular gland and, close to the angle of the mandible, it arches laterally across the stylohyoid and posterior belly of the digastric muscles. It then descends toward the inferior border of the mandible, lying in a groove between the submandibular gland medially and the medial pterygoid muscle laterally. Turning around the inferior border of the mandible, the artery grooves the bone, pierces the superficial cervical fascia, and enters the face at the anterior edge of the masseter muscle.

The *occipital artery* arises from the posterior surface of the external carotid artery, near the level of the facial artery. It passes posteriorly along the inferior border of the posterior belly of the digastric muscle, crosses the anterior surface of the internal jugular vein, and ends in the posterior part of the scalp.

The *posterior auricular artery* is the third branch arising from the posterior wall of the external carotid artery, usually at the superior margin of the posterior belly of the digastric and stylohyoid muscles. It may arise as a common trunk with the occipital artery or as an independent branch. It arches laterally across the stylohyoid muscle, turns posterior, and enters the interval between the posterior margin of the external auditory canal and the mastoid process, where it divides into two terminal branches.

Vagus Nerve

The tenth cranial nerve receives its name from the Latin word *vagus*, which means "wandering." This nerve has the most extensive distribution of all cranial nerves. The vagus nerve leaves the skull through the jugular foramen along with the internal jugular vein and cranial nerves IX and XI. It enters the neck anterior and lateral to the superior cervical ganglion and runs within the carotid sheath between the internal carotid artery and the internal jugular vein in a posterior position (▶ Fig. 2.27).

On the lower part of the right side of the neck, the vagus nerve enters the mediastinum after crossing the origin of the subclavian artery, posterior to the brachiocephalic trunk and the sternoclavicular joint. The right recurrent laryngeal nerve leaves the main trunk of the vagus nerve to loop around the subclavian artery.

On the left side of the neck, the vagus nerve descends between the common carotid and subclavian arteries, anterior to the thoracic duct. In the upper part of the superior mediastinum, the vagus nerve is crossed by the phrenic nerve. In the lower part of the same region it crosses anterior to the root of the subclavian artery and the arch of the aorta. Below the arch of the aorta it passes dorsal to the left main bronchus and divides into branches. The left recurrent nerve loops around the arch of the aorta.

Sympathetic Trunk

The sympathetic trunk runs from the skull base to the subclavian artery lying anterolateral to the vertebral column, posterior to the great vessels, and anterior to the longus colli and longus capitis muscles (▶ Fig. 2.30). It does not receive white rami communicans in the neck, but contains three cervical sympathetic ganglia (superior, medial, and inferior). These ganglia receive their preganglionic fibers from the superior thoracic spinal nerves through white rami communicans, whose fibers leave the spinal cord in the ventral roots of the thoracic spinal nerves. From the sympathetic trunk the fibers pass to cervical structures as postganglionic fibers in cervical spinal nerves, or leave as direct visceral branches.

The *superior cervical ganglion* is the largest of the three cervical sympathetic ganglia. It is located at the level of the atlas and axis, between the internal jugular vein and the internal carotid artery. The carotid sheath lies anterior to the ganglion, and the longus colli muscle is located posterior to it. Postganglionic fibers pass along with the internal carotid artery and enter the cranial cavity. It also sends branches to the external carotid artery and into the four superior cranial nerves.

The *middle cervical ganglion* lies at the level of the cricoid cartilage and the transverse process of C6, anterior to the bend of the inferior thyroid artery. This ganglion may be double or missing entirely. Its postganglionic fibers pass to the thyroid gland and heart.

The *inferior cervical ganglion* lies at the level of the first rib, posterior to the vertebral artery or to the first part of the subclavian artery. It usually fuses with the first thoracic ganglion to form the stellate ganglion or cervicothoracic ganglion. Fibers from this ganglion pass into the vertebral plexus and to the heart.

The sympathetic trunk and its ganglia are located posteriorly to the carotid sheath, enclosed in a splitting of the prevertebral layer of the deep cervical fascia. Damage to the sympathetic trunk in the neck causes Horner syndrome (miosis, ptosis, enophthalmos, and anhidrosis of the ipsilateral eye).

Visceral Compartment of the Neck

The contents of the visceral compartment of the neck are enveloped by the middle layer of the deep cervical fascia. This fascia surrounds the pharynx and cervical esophagus, the larynx and cervical trachea, the thyroid and parathyroid glands, the recurrent laryngeal nerves and the inferior thyroid arteries, along with adipose tissue, lymph nodes and the cranial part of the thymus.

The term *central compartment of the neck* has been reserved during the past decades to define the adipose tissue and lymph nodes that are removed during central neck dissection. It is also known as the level VI of the neck. This includes the pretracheal and paratracheal spaces. The boundaries of the central compartment (▶ Fig. 2.31) are the hyoid bone superiorly, the common carotid arteries laterally, the prevertebral fascia posteriorly, and the strap muscles and superficial layer of the deep cervical fascia anteriorly; inferiorly, the central compartment is continuous with the upper anterior mediastinum, although for surgical purposes an inferior limit has been defined at the level of the innominate artery on the right side, and at a similar level on the left side. The lymph nodes within the central compartment include the following (▶ Fig. 2.5):

2

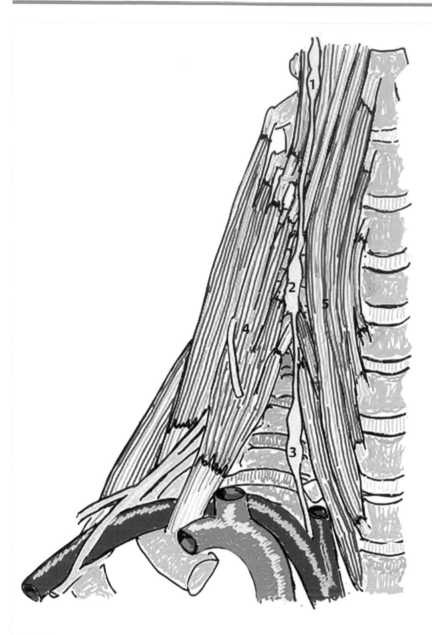

Fig. 2.30 Sympathetic trunk: 1, superior cervical ganglion; 2, middle cervical ganglion; 3, inferior cervical ganglion; 4, scalene muscles; 5, paravertebral muscles.

- Precricoid node: also known as *Delphian node*, as a reference to the Oracle of Delphi because its enlargement was related to bad prognosis of laryngeal cancer. Usually single or double, it is situated anteriorly to the cricothyroid membrane.
- Perithyroidal nodes: a group of inconstant, small, lymph nodes located within the thyroid capsule.
- Pretracheal nodes: in the midline, inferiorly to the thyroid isthmus.
- Paratracheal nodes: at both sides of the cervical trachea, following the course of the recurrent laryngeal nerves.

The *thyroid gland* (▶ Fig. 2.32) is a butterfly-shaped gland. It has two lobes located at both sides of the cervical trachea and larynx, and an isthmus that crosses the anterior wall of the trachea at a variable level, usually on the second, third, and/or fourth tracheal cartilages. The *parathyroid glands* are four small, brown-colored, glands located in the posterior surface of the thyroid lobes. A detailed description of the anatomy of the thyroid and parathyroid glands surpass the purposes of this book.

The *inferior thyroid artery* (▶ Fig. 2.32) is a branch of the thyrocervical trunk, which comes from the subclavian artery. The route of the artery has the shape of a horizontal S. From its origin, it ascends vertically until the level of the sixth cervical vertebra. It then turns medially, crossing the posterior aspect of the common carotid artery to enter the paratracheal space. Immediately, it turns inferiorly and medially for a variable length, and then superiorly again to reach the posterior aspect of the thyroid lobe. The inferior thyroid artery contributes to the irrigation of the thyroid gland, as well as inferior and superior parathyroid glands.

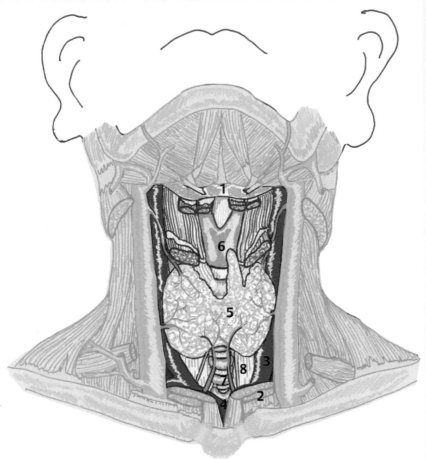

Fig. 2.31 The central compartment of the neck and its limits. 1, hyoid bone; 2, strap muscles; 3, carotid artery; 4, brachiocephalic artery; 5, thyroid gland; 6, larynx; 7, trachea; 8, recurrent laryngeal nerve.

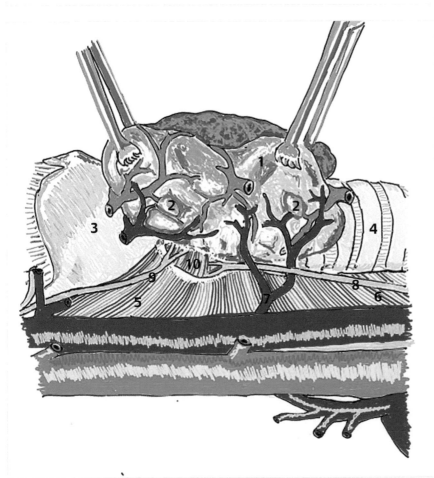

Fig. 2.32 Contents of the central compartment. 1, thyroid gland; 2, parathyroid glands; 3, larynx; 4, trachea; 5, inferior constrictor muscle; 6, esophagus; 7, inferior thyroid artery; 8, recurrent laryngeal nerve; 9, external branch of the superior laryngeal nerve; 10, cricothyroid muscle.

The *recurrent laryngeal nerves* (▶ Fig. 2.32) are the branches of the vagus nerve that innervate most of the intrinsic muscles of the larynx (with the exception of the cricothyroid muscle that is innervated by the external branch of the superior laryngeal nerve). The right recurrent laryngeal nerve emerges off the vagus at the level of the subclavian artery, surrounds this artery, and ascends in an oblique direction from lateral to medial to cross the paratracheal space and enter the larynx. The left recurrent laryngeal nerve originates from the vagus nerve in the mediastinum, at the level of the aortic arch; after surrounding it, the nerve ascends in a more vertical direction than the right one, over the lateral surface of the cervical esophagus or in the trachea-esophageal groove, to reach the larynx. During their course through the paratracheal spaces, both right and left recurrent nerves are related to the posteromedial aspect of the thyroid gland and cross the inferior thyroid artery; the nerves may be superficial to the artery (more frequent on the right side), deep to it (more frequent on the left side), or pass between its terminal branches.

3 The Conceptual Approach to Functional and Selective Neck Dissection

3.1 Introduction

To sum up the essentials of the previous chapters, we may look at the issue of "less than radical" neck dissection under two different standpoints. The American evolution, which is based on the idea of preserving important neck structures that may not be involved by the tumor (e.g., internal jugular vein, spinal accessory nerve, and sterno-cleidomastoid muscle); and the Latin approach, which is based on the fascial concept developed by Osvaldo Suárez.

The end point may be similar but the journey is different.

3.2 Preserving Structures: The American Approach

This approach gave rise to the so-called modified radical neck dissections. After some years of debate, the oncological safety of these "less than radical" operations was finally accepted by all. A step forward in this evolution resulted in the appearance of "selective" neck dissections. In these, some nodal regions are preserved according to the location of the primary tumor. This new approach to neck dissection carried a need for a comprehensive classification inclusive of all types of modifications to the radical operation. Because the potential number of modifications is rather large, the resulting classification is complex and difficult to handle on a daily basis.

3.2.1 Selective Neck Dissections: Types and Indications

Martin objected to the selective approach because it lacked a statistical basis. However, subsequent evidence supports it. The anatomical studies of Rouviere demonstrated that the lymphatic drainage from normal head-and-neck mucosal sites is relatively predictable. Later, clinical studies concluded that oral cavity cancers mostly metastasized to the jugular digastric and midjugular nodes. Cancers of the anterior tongue, floor of the mouth, and buccal mucosa metastasize first to the nodes in the submandibular triangle. Some metastases may skip the submandibular and upper deep jugular nodes and go directly to the midjugular nodes on either side of the neck. The Lindberg study, and a subsequent study by Skolnik, observed that oral cavity and oropharynx tumors rarely metastasize to posterior or lower deep jugular nodes in the absence of metastases in the upper jugular and submaxillary nodal groups. Shah's 1990 retrospective review of radical neck dissection specimens from patients with oral, laryngeal, and pharyngeal cancers concluded that

oral cavity cancers metastasize most often to levels I, II, and III, whereas oropharynx cancers most often go to levels II, III, and IV. When cancerous nodes were found in other levels, they were usually positive in the areas of highest risk too. Bocca and others have observed that supraglottic cancers rarely metastasize to the submental and submandibular nodal groups. Nasopharyngeal and some oropharyngeal tumors can metastasize to the nodes in the posterior triangle of the neck. Finally, subglottic lesions and thyroid malignancies frequently involve the lymph nodes in the anterior central compartment of the neck.

Based on these findings, several selective neck dissections have been proposed. Its classification has varied through years and no terminology has been unanimously adopted. In an effort to standardize it, Ferlito and others in 2011 proposed a classification based on the symbol "ND" for "neck dissection" followed by the nodal groups and nonlymphatic structures removed. However, classic terms such as supraomohyoid, lateral, or posterolateral neck dissection are still common nowadays.

Selective Neck Dissection for Oral Cavity Cancer

The submental, submandibular, upper, and midjugular groups of nodes are the usual sites of metastases from the oral cancers. The term *supraomohyoid neck dissection* includes levels I, II, and III. In the case of invasive oral tongue cancer, including level IV is also recommended. In the absence of clinically evident neck metastases, there is no reason to include level V. Bilateral dissection is recommended for midline tumors (floor of the mouth, ventral surface of the tongue). In patients with significant (N2) nodal metastases in the ipsilateral neck, bilateral dissection or contralateral neck radiation is crucial.

These recommendations suggest that an operation close to a comprehensive functional neck dissection is appropriate for patients with oral cavity cancers with clinically evident metastases, and something less is acceptable for elective dissection. This approach to cancer codifies and structures what experienced surgeons have always done: make intraoperative decisions based on operative findings.

Selective Neck Dissection for Oropharyngeal, Hypopharyngeal, and Laryngeal Cancer

The *lateral neck dissection* is recommended for these sites. It removes nodal groups II, III, and IV, leaving levels I and V undissected. Level IIB is sometimes excluded in laryngeal and hypopharyngeal cancers. The procedure should be done bilaterally in all supraglottic and hypopharyngeal cancers, or if there are proven metastases to one side of the neck. In the case of subglottic or low hypopharyngeal invasion, including level VI is recommended.

Posterolateral Neck Dissection

This operation removes the nodes of levels II, III, IV, and V, the suboccipital, and the postauricular nodal groups. It is recommended for metastases from skin malignancies of the posterior scalp, posterior neck, and some parotid salivary gland cancers that have metastasized posteriorly. The dissection differs from the dissections favored for aerodigestive system metastases. It removes the lymph nodes and lymphatics containing fibrofatty tissue of the posterior neck, the subdermal fat, and fascia between the primary site and nodal compartments where there are no distinct fascial compartments.

Central Compartment Neck Dissection

The term *central compartment* has been widely accepted, and has superseded others like anterior compartment. This dissection removes only area VI, which includes the paratracheal, perithyroid, and precricoid (Delphian) nodes. The procedure is favored for thyroid cancer, cervical trachea, subglottic laryngeal cancer (subglottic or transglottic), cervical esophagus, and hypopharynx cancer. The procedure is usually bilateral for cervical esophageal and large hypopharyngeal cancer. It can be combined with a lateral dissection and occasionally needs to be extended to the upper mediastinum. This selective dissection clarifies the management of an area of potential metastases that has been largely neglected. Nevertheless, there is a dearth of statistical data to make rational decisions about when, how much, whether both sides, when to extend, and so forth. The central compartment dissection seems reasonable because of the definition of its scope.

3.3 Dissecting through Fascial Spaces: The Latin Approach

This approach is based on the anatomical compartmentalization of the neck. The fascial system creates spaces and barriers separating the lymphatic tissue from the remaining neck structures. The lymphatic system of the neck is contained within a fascial envelope, which, under normal conditions, may be removed without taking out other neck structures such as the internal jugular vein, sternocleidomastoid muscle, or spinal accessory nerve. The surgical technique that made this possible was initially referred to as "functional neck dissection" because it allowed a more functional approach to the neck in head-and-neck cancer patients. However, as previously emphasized, the most important but less well-known fact about functional neck dissection is that it represents a surgical

concept with no implications regarding the extent of the surgery. Osvaldo Suárez never performed functional neck dissection as the comprehensive type of neck dissection that some have made of it. In fact, the operation he used for cancer of the larynx did not include the submandibular and submental lymph nodes (area I) in the resection, something that nowadays will be considered a selective neck dissection.

The question that arises at this point is if functional neck dissection was initially designed as a new approach to the neck regardless of the extent of the surgery, why did we make of it just another type of "modified" radical neck dissection? To understand the reasons for this misinterpretation we must take ourselves to the moment when both trends—American and Latin—merged.

The increasing number of reports from European surgeons in the English literature describing the good results obtained with functional neck dissection drew the attention of American surgeons to this procedure. However, the merging of ideas resembled more a collision than a mixture, and the final result was another modification to radical neck dissection. The operation was accepted as an oncologically safe procedure, but the idea was not understood. The battle of functional neck dissection had been won, but the war of the types of neck dissection, the war of the different ways to approach the neck, was lost. To sum up, the real concept of functional neck dissection was lost in translation.

3.4 Functional as a Concept

We are aware that the two approaches herein specified—American and Latin—may look similar to many observers. However, there is a great conceptual difference between them. In the first case the surgical technique is modified to preserve some neck structures, whereas in the second, a different approach is used to treat the neck that has a disease confined to the lymphatic system.

This difference may appear terminological and irrelevant when it comes to comparing "functional" versus "modified radical." It may be said that, although the rationale is different, the end result is the same: the lymphatic system is removed from the neck, preserving the remaining neck structures. However, the situation becomes more complex when selective neck dissections appear in the surgical scenario.

Selective neck dissections are simple modifications of standard operations, whether they are functional or radical (we will see later that they are more closely related to functional than to radical neck dissection). They are just technical variations designed to fit the operation to the patient on a more individualized basis. Thus, their potential number is as high as the number of possible modifications to the original procedure. On the contrary, functional neck dissection as described here is a concept, allowing a different approach to the neck.

The key factor for the misunderstanding of functional neck dissection was the mixture between concepts and techniques that took place in the literature. This situation was favored by a linguistic factor that played an important role in all this confusion.

The functional concept reached the American surgeons through the experience of third parties because Osvaldo Suárez never published his ideas in English. Moreover, the few Spanish papers he published did not emphasize the importance of his approach—as often happens with important contributions, the author is the person least aware of the impact of the innovation. The result of this indirect transmission of information was the partial distortion of the implicit message: functional is a concept, not just another modification.

The functional concept implies dissecting along fascial planes, regardless of the nodal regions that may be preserved or included in the resection. Functional means using fascial compartmentalization to remove the lymphatic tissue of the neck.

The final conclusion for this reasoning is that functional neck dissection should not be identified with a comprehensive type of nonradical neck dissection, but with a conceptual approach to the neck. Whether the surgeon decides to stop above or below the omohyoid muscle in oral cavity tumors, remove or preserve the lymph nodes in the posterior triangle of the neck (lower part of area V) in hypopharyngeal cancer, or resect or spare the submental lymph nodes in laryngeal cancer patients constitutes only minor considerations in regard to the basic principle.

Now let us address the relations between the basic functional principle and selective neck operations.

3.5 Functional and Selective Neck Dissections: So Close and yet So Far

From the information given thus far, it is obvious that the functional concept and the selective operations are more similar than they appear to be in some classifications. They are both indicated for N0 patients, they both preserve neck structures not involved by the tumor, and they both may be performed simultaneously on both sides of the neck. In fact, functional and selective neck dissections are so similar to each other that they could be regarded as the same thing with different names. It is of utmost importance here to understand that the functional concept holds the clue for the oncological safety of all selective neck dissections.

If functional neck dissection is a concept, selective operations are the materialization of this concept. Thus, the functional concept includes in its definition all types of selective neck dissections because they all share the same rationale and indications of the functional approach. The differences between the various selective operations are

only technical considerations emerging from a common, standard comprehensive functional neck dissection.

One of the advantages of this conceptual approach to nonradical neck dissection is that it provides the rationale for the oncological safety of selective neck dissections. On the other hand, a conceptual approach like this reduces the relative importance of selective neck dissections, which are now regarded not as different operations, but as technical variations of the original procedure.

3.6 Reasons for the Oncological Safety of Selective Neck Dissections

Fascial compartmentalization of the neck provides the oncological safety for selective neck dissections by the inclusion of lymph nodes and ducts in a system of fascial spaces and barriers. It is possible to remove the lymphatic system without removing other neck structures as long as the tumor cells remain within the lymph node capsule.

The decision of whether to remove the whole lymphatic system of the neck or just a part of it will depend on several factors, including the location of the primary tumor, the N stage, and the experience and preferences of the surgeon.

The distribution of cervical lymph node metastases from head-and-neck tumors has been a matter of study and debate over many years. Nowadays we have a fairly consistent description of the most frequent metastatic areas for most primary sites in the head and neck. This situation allows the surgeon to preserve some nodal groups according to the location of the primary tumor without a significant risk of undertreatment. This is especially true in pathological N0 patients in whom the lymph flow should not have been disturbed by metastatic disease. However, in pN+ necks the situation may be different. Two problems must be considered in patients with metastatic disease in the lymphatic system of the neck:

1. The theoretical predictability of the lymph node metastatic pattern may have been modified by changes produced by the tumor cells contained within the lymphatic system. This may result in positive nodes outside the "normal" route. These nodes will be missed by a selective operation that otherwise could have been safe.

2. The presence of metastasis in the usual nodal areas significantly increases the chances for positive nodes in other less frequent regions for the primary site. In the preoperative clinically N+ neck with small palpable nodes, this is the strongest argument against selective neck dissections. In these patients, a comprehensive functional neck dissection must be performed to include all the lymphatic systems of the neck. The problem is different in the clinically N0 neck treated with selective neck dissection in which occult

metastases are diagnosed after the operation. In these cases, selective neck dissection may be regarded as a staging rather than a therapeutic operation, and postoperative radiotherapy may be needed.

This is one of the strongest arguments against the use of super-selective operations because the surgeon never knows before surgery which patients will show positive nodes at pathology after the operation. From the patient perspective, assuming the risk for a smaller operation is only justified on the basis of improved oncological results and decreased morbidity. The first criterion, oncological safety, has only been demonstrated for a small number of selective operations. On the other hand, decreased morbidity is at least questionable when it comes to comparing the results of comprehensive functional neck dissection with those of the most frequently recommended selective procedures. It is not preservation of lymphatic regions but of nonlymphatic structures that is related to surgical morbidity and sequelae in neck dissection.

The previous considerations support the important role that personal experience of the surgeon ultimately plays in selecting the type of dissection that should be used for different primary head-and-neck tumors. And personal experience is acquired only after years of practice with standard procedures and sound apprehension of fundamental concepts.

In conclusion, whereas the oncological safety of some selective neck dissections has already been proved, the feasibility of others still lacks sound scientific demonstration and should be documented by means of well-designed trials. While we wait for the confirmation of the oncological safety of these procedures, it is our policy to teach basic concepts rather than technical modifications in the hope that time and experience will allow well-trained surgeons to adequately adjust their operations to the best interest of their patients.

3.7 The Role of Selective Neck Dissections in the Functional Approach

In the functional approach, a selective neck dissection (SND) is just a technical modification of the complete operation, which includes all nodal regions in the resection. We do not question the usefulness of these operations. In fact, a large number of our nonradical operations are selective neck dissections. However, we do not share the need to establish a comprehensive classification that includes all possible types of modifications and technical variations. The number of combinations and permutations of nine nodal regions and subregions along with more than 10 primary sites, plus two preoperative N stages, is immense. Such classification is impractical for teaching purposes.

Some authors support the need to create extensive classifications as a tool to obtain proper information about the usefulness of different types of selective neck dissection. However, the validity of such reasoning is questionable. The ill-defined boundaries that delineate the separation of nodal regions at surgery stand as an important drawback for standardizing purposes. Although clearly marked in theory, the anatomical landmarks that separate the nodal groups are difficult to identify during the operation. The artificial lines that divide the neck into nodal regions are not easily visible and the anatomical landmarks that may be used to help the surgeon can be largely displaced during the operative maneuvers. This gives little consistency to the reports of selective neck dissections coming from different institutions, and even from different surgeons within the same institution. What somebody refers to as SND (II–IV) may be different in extension, number of removed lymph nodes, and true anatomical boundaries to the SND (II–IV) performed by other surgeons. Extending this situation to all types of selective neck dissections gives an idea of the actual inconsistency of the current classification from a practical standpoint.

3.8 Neck Dissection Classifications: Making Complex What Is Simple

Classifications reflect the human desire to understand the complexity of our environment and make it easier to be managed. Unfortunately, very often, the classification is even more complex than the reality. This is the case with neck dissection.

For a neck dissection there are two ways to approach the neck: functional and radical. You can substitute these two names with those of your preference, but the concept remains the same.

With "functional" you approach the neck driving your knife through the fascial planes. You remove the fibrofatty tissue containing the lymphatic system of the neck by pealing it from the surrounding structures just taking your dissection over the fascia of the neck. This approach is only possible when the tumor is confined within the boundaries of the lymph nodes. Surgery is directed against the lymphatic system that contains the tumor.

With "radical" you approach the neck in a "cross-country" fashion. No planes are searched. Cuts are made up, down, medial, and lateral, and all the contents of the neck are removed with the exception of the carotid artery. This aggressive approach is required when the tumor spreads out of the lymphatic tissue and invades the adjacent structures (muscles, veins, nerves, glands). Here, the surgery is directed against the neck that has been invaded by the tumor.

These two approaches do not have anything to do with the extent of the dissection. The limits of our surgery will

Table 3.1 Commonly used classifications of neck dissection

AAO–HNS 2002	1. Radical neck dissection 2. Modified radical neck dissection 3. Selective neck dissection Each variation is depicted by SND and levels removed, e.g., SND (I, II, III, and IV) 4. Extended neck dissection
AHNS–AAOHNS 2008	1. Incorporates sublevels 2. Acknowledges the term *total ND* 3. Incorporates radiological landmarks 4. Redefines boundary between Ib and IIa—SMG 5. Defines lymph node group VII 6. Emphasizes pathological analysis

Ferlito et al 2011, *Head and Neck*	Proposed nomenclature	AAO-NHS/AHNS equivalence
	ND (I–V, SCM, IJV, CN XI)	Radical neck dissection
	ND (I–V, SCM, IJV, CN XI, and CN XII)	Extended neck dissection with removal of the hypoglossal nerve
	ND (I–V, SCM, IJV)	Modified radical neck dissection with preservation of the spinal accessory nerve
	ND (II–IV)	Selective neck dissection (II–IV)
	ND (II–IV, VI)	Selective neck dissection (II–IV, VI)
	ND (II–IV, SCM)	NA
	ND (I–III)	Selective neck dissection (I–III)
	ND (I–III, SCM, IJV, CN XI)	NA
	ND (II, III)	Selective neck dissection (II, III)
	ND (IIA, III)	Selective neck dissection (IIA, III)
	ND (VI)	Selective neck dissection (VI)
	ND (VI, VII)	Selective neck dissection (VI, VII)

Abbreviations: ND, neck dissection; SND, selective neck dissection; SCM, sternocleidomastoid muscle; SMG, submandibular gland; IJV, internal jugular vein; CN, cranial nerve; NA, not available.

depend on many factors. With the radical approach, it is easier to imagine the surgical boundaries. These patients usually have large neck masses that make aggressive resections necessary.

The problem comes when we deal with the "functional" approach. Here the extent of the dissection depends on many factors. Some are tumor-related (site, stage) while others are of a different kind (morbidity, cost, reimbursement issues). This diversity is what makes neck dissection classification so complex. Some examples are shown in ▶ Table 3.1. In our opinion, the newer the classification is, the more impractical it seems.

For teaching purposes we prefer to use a more pragmatic approach that includes only two different types of neck dissection that represent the two main concepts: functional and radical (▶ Table 3.2). After the young surgeons have learned the basics of these two approaches, they will decide whether to extend their practice with technical modifications to the standard procedures, based on their personal experience. An additional group of modified procedures is included in our classification for special situations. We accept the criticism of those who consider this to be a very simplistic approach to neck dissection classification. Those supporting more detailed classifications consider our approach to be inadequate for comparison purposes between different surgeons and institutions. However, in our opinion, exhaustive

Table 3.2 Conceptual classification of neck dissection used for teaching purposes

Functional neck dissection	Neck dissection following the anatomical fascial planes defined by fascial compartmentalization of the neck *The extension of the dissection will depend on the location of the primary tumor and the experience of the surgeon. Surgical details should be reported at the end of the operation*
Radical neck dissection	Neck dissection according to the guidelines described by Crile in 1906 and popularized later by Martin *The extension of the dissection will depend on the location of the primary tumor and the experience of the surgeon. Surgical details should be reported at the end of the operation*
Modified neck dissections	
Modified functional neck dissection	Fascial neck dissection, including the resection of one or more nonlymphatic structures usually preserved in conventional functional neck dissection (internal jugular vein, sternocleidomastoid muscle, spinal accessory nerve)[a]
Modified radical neck dissection	Neck dissection performed according to the surgical principles of the Crile operation, with preservation of one or more nonlymphatic structures usually removed in radical neck dissection (internal jugular vein, sternocleidomastoid muscle, spinal accessory nerve)[a]

[a]The surgical report must detail the resected structure(s).

classifications do not allow useful comparisons as a consequence of the multiple subjective variables that take part in every operation, especially when the surgical limits are diffuse and difficult to identify. In contrast to simpler systems, exhaustive systems are more difficult to learn and use in everyday life.

On the other hand, for clinical purposes we frequently use selective neck dissections, but only those that have been proved safe in our hands over the years (e.g., preserving level I in cancer of the larynx). However, we consider them simple modifications of the standard procedures and do not pay special attention to nomenclature and other terminological issues. Each one of these operations is selected on a personal basis according to factors relating to the primary tumor, the patient, and the treatment team. This selection process results in a polymorphous variety of procedures designed to fit the operation to the patient on a personal basis.

It must be emphasized that we never push the limits too far concerning the preservation of nodal regions. There are two reasons for this: (1) the wish to avoid "staging" operations when therapeutic procedures are easily achievable and (2) the belief that the time and morbidity added with more extensive operations are not significant from the patient's perspective. With this approach we try to increase the effectiveness of our surgery and limit the need for postoperative radiotherapy in early N stages, reducing the cost and morbidity of the treatment.

3.9 Indications and Limitations of the Functional Approach

To be safe, functional neck surgery requires all metastatic disease to be confined within the lymphatic tissue. Thus, this approach is ideal for N0 patients with a high risk of occult metastasis. An additional advantage of functional neck dissection is that it may be performed simultaneously on both sides of the neck without increasing morbidity. In all midline head-and-neck lesions with high risk of cervical metastasis (floor of the mouth, base of the tongue, supraglottic larynx), functional neck dissection is the best surgical option for N0 patients.

In patients with small palpable nodes, functional neck dissection is still a valid option as long as some principles are carefully observed. The nodes should not be greater than 2.5 to 3.0 cm in greatest diameter. This is justified by the need to have all metastatic disease confined within the lymph node capsule. Although extracapsular spread is possible in lymph nodes of all sizes, it is well known that extracapsular spread increases with increasing lymph node size. Gross extracapsular extension results in lymph node fixation to contiguous structures. Therefore, lymph node mobility must be carefully assessed before and during surgery. This is even more important than the absolute size in centimeters because small nodes may be fixed, thus preventing a functional approach in these cases. In no instance should functional neck dissection be attempted in patients with fixed nodes. If at surgery there is any doubt about the feasibility of the functional operation, the suspicious structure (vein, muscle, gland, or nerve) must be removed with the specimen. Cancer cells cannot be pursued with a scalpel, and surgical demonstrations of "technical expertise" are unacceptable in cancer patients and must be reserved for the dissection room.

The number of palpable nodes is not a contraindication for functional neck dissection as long as all nodes fulfill the previously mentioned criteria. The same can be said with respect to the location of the primary tumor. Functional neck dissection is as safe for supraglottic tumor as it is for piriform sinus cancer, as long as the indications are carefully followed in both situations. The fact that patients with cancer of the hypopharynx do worse than those with laryngeal tumors cannot be modified by performing more aggressive operations than those required for the N stage of the patient.

By definition, functional neck dissection is not possible in patients previously treated with radiotherapy or other types of neck surgery. In these patients the fascial planes have disappeared as a consequence of the previous treatment. Thus, fascial dissection is not possible anymore. In these cases modified radical neck dissection appears as an alternative to radical neck dissection as a means to preserve structures not involved by the tumor. The dissection will be made according to the basic principles of radical neck dissection, but preservation of uninvolved neck structures will be accomplished according to the surgical scenario. This is a clear example that illustrates the difference between functional and modified radical neck dissection.

4 Surgical Technique

4.1 Introduction

This chapter describes the surgical technique for a complete functional approach to the neck in which all cervical nodal groups are removed. For teaching purposes, the surgical steps are sequentially detailed. However, not every single surgical step of those mentioned must be considered mandatory for every malignant head-and-neck tumor. As previously emphasized in this book, the preservation of selected nodal groups is a valid option that does not modify the basic principle of the functional approach to the neck (i.e., the removal of lymphatic tissue by means of fascial dissection). Surgeons must be able to decide, according to their own personal experience, which nodal groups should be included in the dissection and which can be preserved, then proceed accordingly, skipping the surgical steps that may not be considered necessary.

4.2 Preoperative Preparation and Operating Room Setup

The patient should be prepared as for any major operation. Preoperative evaluation is accomplished by the anesthesiologist prior to surgery. Premedication is used according to the anesthesiologist's choice. Prophylactic antibiotics are given according to the usual protocol. The patient's neck and upper chest are shaved and prepared for the operation.

The patient is placed supine on the operating table with a roll or inflatable rubber bag under the shoulders to obtain the proper angle for surgery (▶ Fig. 4.1). This is generally obtained when the occiput rests against the upper end of the table. Elevating the upper half of the operating table to approximately 30 degrees will decrease the amount of bleeding during surgery. A bloodless field will decrease the operating time and help the identification of neck structures.

The patient's lower face, ears, neck, shoulders, and upper chest are prepared with surgical solution, and the patient is draped in layers (▶ Fig. 4.2). Four towels are placed and affixed to the skin. Two of the towels are placed horizontally, one from the chin to the mastoid over the body of the mandible and the other across the upper chest from the shoulder to the midline. The remaining two towels are placed vertically, from the mastoid tip to the shoulder, except for unilateral procedures where the second vertical towel is placed in the midline. A sheet is placed over the patient's chest and legs, and an open sheet covers the entire patient except for the field of operation. The Mayo stand is secured to the operating table over the thighs of the patient (▶ Fig. 4.3).

Two assistants are usually present: one in front of the surgeon and the second at the patient's head. The scrub nurse stands on the right side of the patient facing the head of the table. The ventilator and the anesthetist are placed on the left side of the patient (▶ Fig. 4.4). Few general instruments are needed for the operation (▶ Fig. 4.5).

Muscular relaxation is usually avoided to perceive muscle contraction when approaching the main nerves of the neck, especially the spinal-accessory nerve. A nerve stimulator may be useful, although not necessary. We do

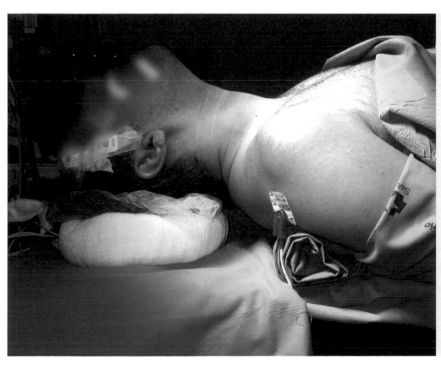

Fig. 4.1 Patient prepared for surgery: a roll is placed under the shoulders to obtain adequate neck extension, and the head is fitted onto a cotton donut to prevent involuntary rotations during the procedure.

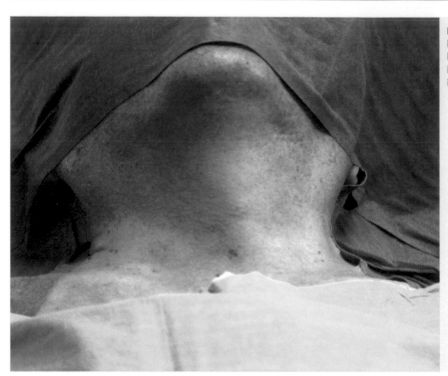

Fig. 4.2 The patient is covered with drapes for a bilateral neck dissection. Superiorly, the inferior border of the mandible and the tip of the ear lobes (mastoids) are seen. The clavicles mark the inferior limit.

not routinely perform intraoperative monitoring of the vagus nerve with endolaryngeal electrodes, except when the procedure involves the thyroid gland and the recurrent laryngeal nerve must be identified and preserved.

4.3 Incision and Flaps

The exact location and type of skin incision will depend on the site of the primary tumor and whether a unilateral or bilateral neck dissection is planned. The following are the main goals to be achieved by the skin incision:
- Allow adequate exposure of the surgical field.
- Assure adequate vascularization of the skin flaps.
- Protect the carotid artery if the sternocleidomastoid muscle must be sacrificed.
- Include scars from previous procedures (e.g., surgery and biopsy).
- Consider the location of the primary tumor.
- Facilitate the use of reconstructive techniques.
- Contemplate the potential need of postoperative radiotherapy.
- Produce acceptable cosmetic results.

A popular incision in our practice is the classic *Gluck-Sorenson* incision (▶ Fig. 4.6a), which is basically an apron flap incision. It starts on the mastoid tip, descends vertically through the sternocleidomastoid muscle to the supraclavicular area, and turns medially to cross the midline; the incision is prolonged contralaterally in a symmetrical fashion on bilateral procedures. The incision must be carried along the posterior border of the sternocleidomastoid muscle to facilitate the approach of the

supraclavicular area when the lymph nodes in this region have to be removed. This incision allows good exposure when the neck dissection is to be combined with a laryngectomy or a thyroidectomy. When the operation includes a total laryngectomy, the midline is crossed a few centimeters above the suprasternal notch, and the stoma is usually incorporated in the incision. On the other hand, for partial laryngectomies and other tumors requiring temporary tracheostomy, the incision crosses the midline at the level of the cricoid cartilage and a small independent horizontal incision can be made at the level of the tracheostomy.

The *single-Y* incision (▶ Fig. 4.6b) is common in our practice for unilateral functional and selective neck dissection that includes the submandibular area and does not need a laryngectomy or a thyroidectomy (e.g., for oropharyngeal cancer). It is also useful when the removal of the primary tumor requires transmandibular approach, which may be accomplished by a chin and labial extension. A well-known disadvantage of this incision is the compromise to the blood supply, especially in the crossing of the incision. Thus, the vertical arm of the incision should be placed posterior to the carotid artery. The cosmetic result is improved by giving the vertical arm a slightly S-shaped curve.

Many other skin incisions have been described and may be used depending on the clinical characteristics of the lesion and the personal preference of the surgeon.

After the incision is completed, the skin flaps are elevated deep to the platysma muscle, preserving the superficial layer of the cervical fascia (▶ Fig. 4.7). Preservation of the external lymphatic envelope allows further fulfillment of the basic anatomical principle of the functional

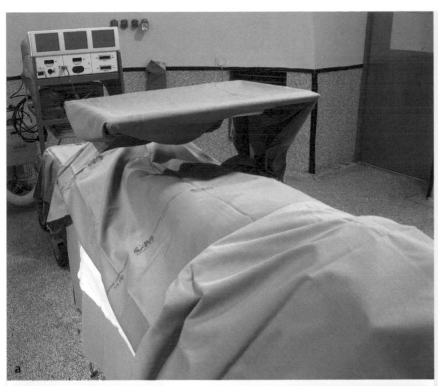

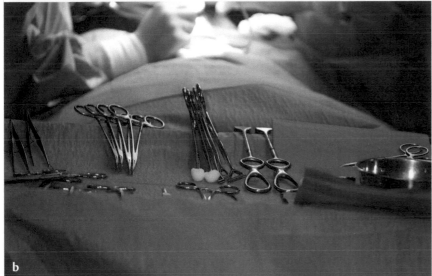

Fig. 4.3 (a) Mayo stand located over the patient's thighs. The scrub nurse will be standing in front of the stand, at the right side of the surgeon. (b) Surgical view from the Mayo stand with the most common instruments on it, ready to be served to the surgeon.

4

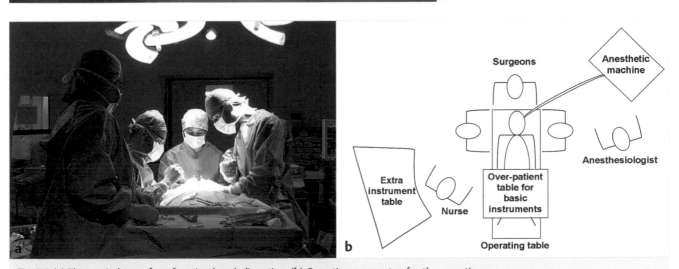

Fig. 4.4 (a) The surgical team for a functional neck dissection. (b) Operating room setup for the operation.

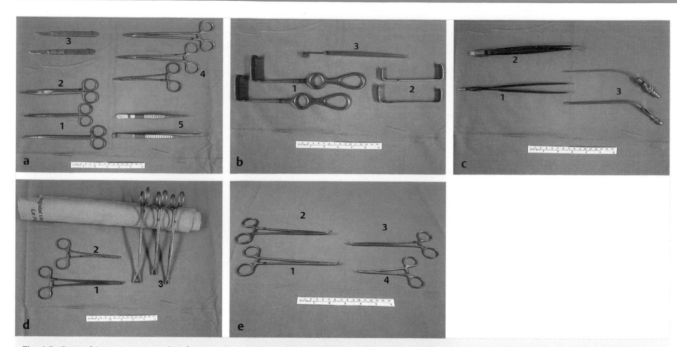

Fig. 4.5 General instruments used in functional and selective neck dissection. (a) 1, curve dissecting scissors; 2, Mayo scissors (to cut threads); 3, knives (#10, #15); 4, needle holders; 5, atraumatic tissue forceps. (b) 1, Langenbeck retractors (to retract superiorly digastric muscle); 2, Farabeuf retractors (to retract laterally sternocleidomastoid muscle); 3, Desmarres vascular retractor (to retract internal jugular vein when needed). (c) 1, monopolar coagulation forceps; 2, bipolar coagulation forceps; 3, suction tips. (d) 1, large Allis forceps (we include two of them in each set, to hold gauze balls); 2, small Allis forceps (we include 15 of them in each set, to grasp fat and other tissues); 3, Duval forceps (we include one large, one medium, and one small in each set, to grasp thyroid gland). (e) 1, right-angle forceps (to ligate internal jugular vein when needed); 2, curved Pean forceps (to ligate thyroid isthmus when needed); 3, curved hemostatic forceps (we include 10 of them in each set, to ligate large vessels and to grasp fascias); 4, mosquito forceps (we include 10 of them in each set, to ligate small vessels).

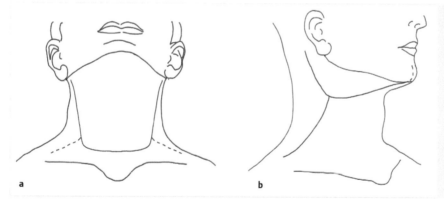

Fig. 4.6 Some popular skin incisions for functional and selective neck dissection. (a) Gluck-Sorenson incision. (b) Single-Y incision.

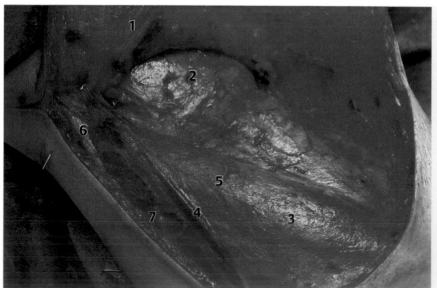

Fig. 4.7 The skin flaps have been raised, preserving the superficial layer of the deep cervical fascia (right side of the neck). 1, upper skin flap; 2, submandibular gland; 3, sternocleidomastoid muscle; 4, external jugular vein; 5, transverse cervical branch from the superficial cervical plexus; 6, great auricular nerve; 7, Erb's point.

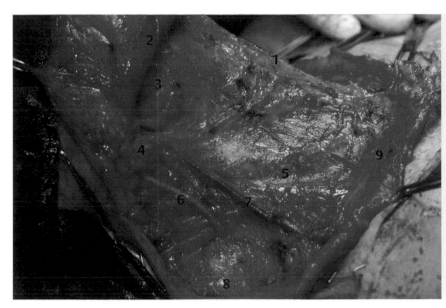

Fig. 4.8 Boundaries of a complete functional neck dissection on the right side of the neck. 1, midline; 2, inferior border of the mandible; 3, submandibular gland; 4, tail of the parotid gland; 5, sternocleidomastoid muscle; 6, great auricular nerve; 7, external jugular vein; 8, trapezius muscle; 9, clavicle.

approach (i.e., the removal of the fascial walls of the lymphatic container along with the lymphatic tissue of the neck).

The limits for a comprehensive functional neck dissection are similar to those of the classic radical neck dissection (▶ Fig. 4.8). The surgical field should expose superiorly the inferior border of the mandible and the tail of the parotid gland. Inferiorly, the flap should be raised up to the level of the clavicle and the sternal notch. The midline of the neck will be the anterior border of the surgical field for a unilateral neck dissection. Finally, the great auricular nerve and the posterior border of the sternocleidomastoid muscle in the upper part of the surgical field, and the anterior border of the trapezius muscle in the lower half of the neck, constitute the posterior boundary of the dissection. After the flaps have been raised, the underlying neck structures can be seen shining through the superficial layer of the cervical fascia (▶ Fig. 4.7, ▶ Fig. 4.8).

The skin flaps must be protected by suturing wet surgical sponges on their internal borders (▶ Fig. 4.9). Pulling from these sponges will help to create tension to the tissues during the procedure. Frequent moistening of the sponges will help to keep the skin flaps in good condition throughout the operation. It should be remembered that this may be a long operation since neck dissection is often performed in conjunction with removal of the primary tumor and, in some instances, reconstructive procedures. Thus, all efforts should be made to preserve the skin in good condition until the end of the procedure.

4.4 Dissection of the Sternocleidomastoid Muscle

Usually, the first step of the operation is the dissection of the fascia that covers the sternocleidomastoid muscle. The goal of this maneuver is to completely unwrap the muscle from its surrounding fascia.

The external jugular vein must be transected during the dissection of the fascia of the sternocleidomastoid muscle. Thus, prior to approaching the fascia, the external jugular vein is usually ligated and divided to facilitate the following maneuvers. Usually, two sections of the external jugular vein are required in functional and selective neck dissection at this stage (▶ Fig. 4.10): (1) at the posterior border of the sternocleidomastoid muscle, right inferiorly to Erb's point; and (2) at the tail of the parotid gland, where the external jugular vein begins by the union of the retromandibular and posterior auricular veins. The external jugular vein should be ligated and divided at a third point at a later step of the operation, within the posterior triangle of the neck when this nodal region is included in the dissection.

The dissection of the sternocleidomastoid muscle begins with a longitudinal incision over the fascia, along the entire length of the muscle. This cut is made with a number-10 knife blade and must be placed near the posterior border of the muscle (▶ Fig. 4.11). The stroke of the knife runs parallel and immediately anterior to the great auricular nerve in the upper half, transects the transverse cervical nerve and the external jugular vein (ligated and divided on a previous step), and follows the posterior border of the muscle in the inferior half. This facilitates the dissection of the sternocleidomastoid muscle because the cleavage plane between the fascia and the muscle is much easier to identify in a forward direction. The external jugular vein is included in the specimen and dissected forward with the fascia of the sternocleidomastoid muscle (▶ Fig. 4.12). Using several hemostats, one of the assistants retracts the fascia medially while the surgeon carries the dissection toward the anterior margin of the muscle. Fascial retraction should be done with extreme care because

4

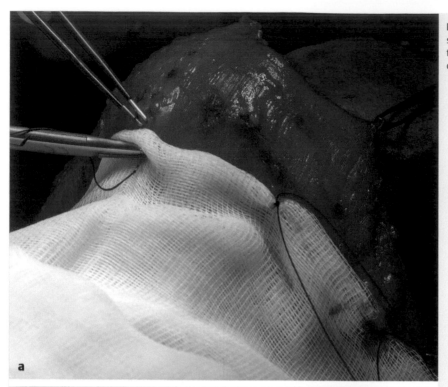

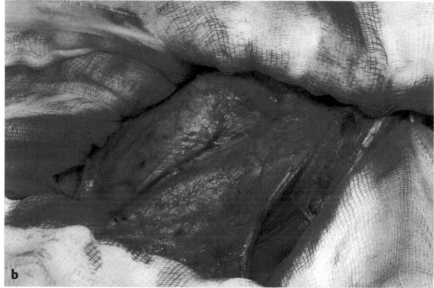

Fig. 4.9 (a,b) Surgical sponges are sutured to the skin flaps to protect them and to help create tension. Keep these sponges wet during the operation.

the thin superficial layer of the cervical fascia is the only tissue now included in the specimen.

We strongly recommend performing this, as well as most other parts of the operation, using knife dissection. The fascial planes of the neck are mainly avascular and can be easily followed with the scalpel. For knife dissection to be most effective the tissue must be under traction. An important task of the assistants throughout the operation is to apply adequate pressure to the dissected tissue.

When the dissection reaches the anterior border of the sternocleidomastoid muscle, the hemostats that have been used to retract the fascia may be left lying on the medial

part of the surgical field hanging toward the opposite side. This will maintain the required amount of traction while freeing the assistants' hands. Further tension may be applied with a hand and a gauze. Then the muscle is retracted posteriorly to continue the dissection over its medial face. Retraction may be performed by the assistant sited at the head of the patient; or by the main surgeon, while holding the knife with the other hand (▶ Fig. 4.13).

Until this point, the cleavage plane between the muscle and the fascia is avascular. However, when the deep medial face of the muscle is approached, small perforating vessels are found entering the muscle through the fascia

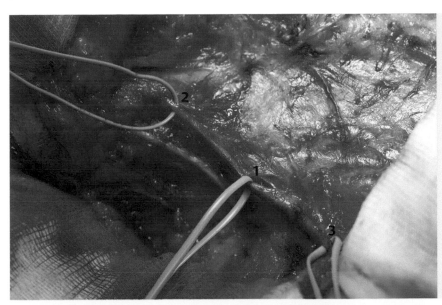

Fig. 4.10 Points of division of the external jugular vein on a right functional neck dissection. 1, posterior border of the sternocleidomastoid muscle; 2, tail of the parotid gland; 3, supraclavicular fossa.

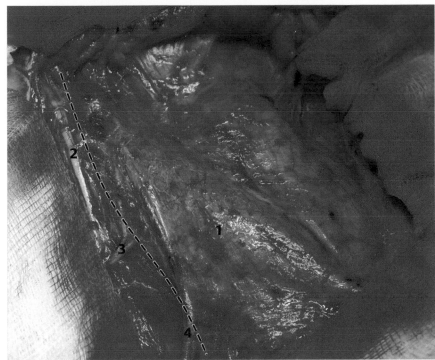

Fig. 4.11 Incision of the fascia over the sternocleidomastoid muscle on the right side of the neck (dashed line). 1, sternocleidomastoid muscle; 2, great auricular nerve; 3, transverse cervical nerve; 4, external jugular vein.

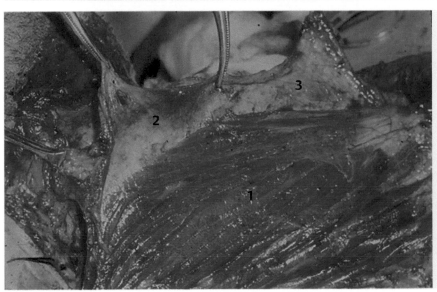

Fig. 4.12 The fascia of the sternocleidomastoid muscle is dissected medially. The external jugular vein is included in the fascia (right side of the neck). 1, sternocleidomastoid muscle; 2, fascia; 3, external jugular vein.

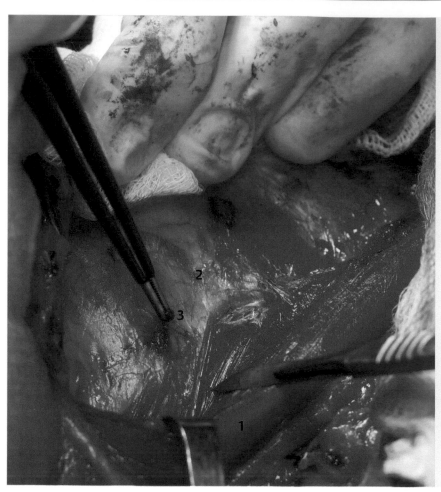

Fig. 4.13 Lateral retraction of the sternocleidomastoid muscle allows the dissection of the medial surface of the muscle. The assistant pulls medially of the dissected fascia with one hand to keep tension, while coagulates the vessels with the other hand.
1, sternocleidomastoid muscle; 2, dissected fascia; 3, vessel to the deep face of the muscle (divided and coagulated).

(▸ Fig. 4.13). The assistant must now cauterize the vessels while the surgeon continues the dissection over the entire medial surface of the sternocleidomastoid muscle. The surgeon must be extremely careful at the upper half of this region, where the spinal accessory nerve enters the muscle. One or more small vessels usually accompany the spinal accessory nerve, which often divides before entering the muscle. The vessels should be cauterized without injuring the nerve, and all branches of the nerve must be preserved to obtain the best shoulder function. More details concerning the dissection of the spinal accessory nerve are given on a later stage of the operation.

After all the small vessels entering the sternocleidomastoid muscle have been cauterized, a new avascular fascial plane is entered and the dissection continues posteriorly along the entire length of the muscle. The internal jugular vein can now be seen through the fascia of the carotid sheath (▸ Fig. 4.14).

The muscle is now almost completely separated from its covering fascia except for a small portion at the posterior border. This part of the muscle will be dissected on a later stage of the procedure. Wet surgical sponges are now introduced in the lower half of the sternocleidomastoid muscle, between the muscle and its dissected fascia. They will serve two purposes: (1) maintain the desired

moisture of the dissected tissues while the attention shifts to the upper part of the surgical field; and (2) serve as a reference for the dissection of the fascia that still covers the posterior border of the sternocleidomastoid muscle, on a later stage of the operation.

The surgeon now moves to the upper part of the surgical field to complete the identification of the spinal accessory nerve. For a better understanding of the following steps of the operation, at this point it may help the reader to take a short pause in the technical details to realize how the surgical approach is made with respect to the sternocleidomastoid muscle when the posterior triangle is included in the resection.

4.5 Management of the Sternocleidomastoid Muscle

A comprehensive dissection of the posterior triangle of the neck is facilitated by a combined approach, both posterior and anterior to the sternocleidomastoid muscle (▸ Fig. 4.15). In the upper half of the neck the dissection is performed anterior to the sternocleidomastoid muscle, whereas in the lower half of the neck the supraclavicular fossa is approached posterior to the sternocleidomastoid muscle.

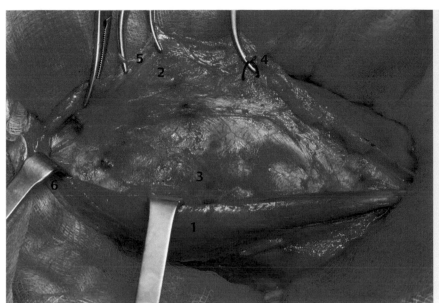

Fig. 4.14 The dissection of the medial face of the sternocleidomastoid muscle has been completed (right side of the neck). 1, sternocleidomastoid muscle; 2, dissected fascia; 3, internal jugular vein (shining through the fascia); 4, external jugular vein (ligated and divided); 5, transverse cervical nerve (divided); 6, great auricular nerve (preserved).

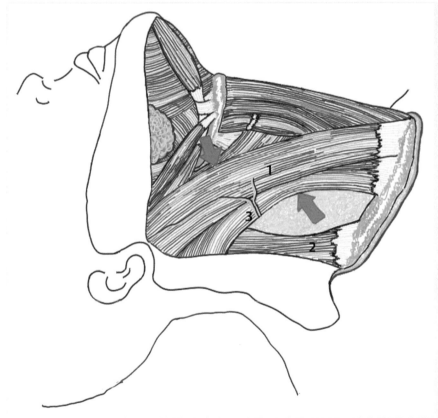

Fig. 4.15 Schematic view of the approach to the neck for a comprehensive functional neck dissection. Above Erb's point the operation is performed anterior to the sternocleidomastoid muscle. The lower part of the posterior triangle (supraclavicular fossa) is approached posterior to the sternocleidomastoid muscle.
1, sternocleidomastoid muscle; 2, trapezius muscle; 3, Erb's point.

To better understand this, imagine the surgical field divided in two halves by a plane passing through Erb's point, the place where the superficial branches of the cervical plexus appear at the posterior border of the sternocleidomastoid muscle. This creates an upper and a lower part of the neck.

The upper half of this division includes the submental and submandibular nodes (area I), the upper part of the posterior triangle of the neck (upper part of area V), and part of the lymphatic chain of the internal jugular vein (area II and part of area III). The dissection of the upper half of this division is performed anteriorly to the sternocleidomastoid muscle. For this purpose, the muscle must be retracted posteriorly throughout the dissection.

The lower half of this imaginary division includes the supraclavicular fossa (lower part of area V), the lower part

4

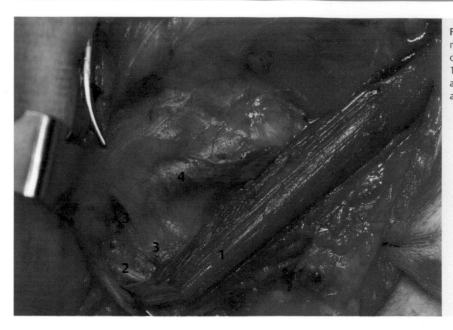

Fig. 4.16 Identification of the spinal accessory nerve during the dissection of the medial surface of the sternocleidomastoid muscle.
1, sternocleidomastoid muscle; 2, spinal accessory nerve; 3, satellite vessel (coagulated and divided); 4, internal jugular vein.

of the lymphatic chain of the internal jugular vein (area IV and part of area III), and the paratracheal lymph nodes (area VI). These regions will be approached both posterior and anterior to the sternocleidomastoid muscle. The supraclavicular fossa will be dissected from behind the muscle, and the remaining lymph structures of the lower half of the neck will be approached anterior to the sternocleidomastoid muscle.

For the surgical specimen to be removed en bloc, the tissue removed from the supraclavicular fossa will be passed beneath the sternocleidomastoid muscle to meet the remaining part of the specimen.

This maneuver, which has always been difficult to understand, may also be performed anterior to the sternocleidomastoid muscle by strong posterior retraction of the muscle. Thus, the lower part of area V can be approached anterior to the sternocleidomastoid muscle and removed with the rest of the specimen in cases where the location of the primary tumor requires complete removal of the supraclavicular fibrofatty tissue (area V).

Now we shall resume the dissection at the point where we left it. The sternocleidomastoid muscle was almost completely free of its fascia, except for a small part at the posterior edge of the muscle, and the attention of the surgeon was directed to the upper part of the surgical field to identify the spinal accessory nerve on its course between the jugular foramen and the sternocleidomastoid muscle.

4.6 Identification of the Spinal Accessory Nerve

The main goal of this step of the operation is to identify the nerve at the entrance of the sternocleidomastoid muscle. This maneuver is helpful to avoid injuring the nerve while dissecting the fascia of the upper part of the

sternocleidomastoid muscle and should be performed before completing the former step. The dissection of the entire course of the nerve between the sternocleidomastoid muscle and the internal jugular vein will be performed in a later step of the procedure.

The spinal accessory nerve enters the sternocleidomastoid muscle approximately at the junction of the upper and middle third of the muscle (▶ Fig. 4.16). Adequate exposure of the area requires posterior retraction of the sternocleidomastoid muscle. The small vessels that usually go along with the nerve are carefully cauterized and the nerve is examined for divisions that may appear before it enters the muscle. All nerve branches must be preserved to obtain the best shoulder function. Sometimes a branch from the second cervical nerve can be seen joining the spinal accessory nerve before its entrance into the sternocleidomastoid muscle. Although most anatomy books consider this and other branches from the cervical plexus to be mainly sensory, it is our experience that preservation of these branches helps to prevent shoulder dysfunction after the operation.

Once the nerve is identified, wet surgical sponges are introduced between the muscle and the fascia, avoiding excessive pressure and stretching maneuvers that may lead to spinal accessory nerve damage. The dissection now continues along the upper limit of the surgical field.

4.7 Dissection of the Submandibular Fossa

From a technical standpoint, a comprehensive removal of the submental and submandibular lymph nodes (area I) is aided by removing the submandibular gland. However, many tumors, such as cancer of the larynx, hypopharynx, or thyroid gland, usually do not require the dissection of level I, and the gland may be preserved. In fact, preservation of the submandibular gland was originally described by Osvaldo Suárez as one of the advantages of the functional approach to the neck. The following description will present the surgical details of submandibular and submental lymph node removal (area I), including the resection of the submandibular gland (for technical details concerning submandibular gland preservation, see Chapter 5).

Dissection of the submandibular and submental triangle starts with a fascial incision along the upper boundary of the surgical field, from the midline to the tail of the parotid gland. The fascia is incised at the submental area and the tissue in the submental region is dissected inferiorly (▶ Fig. 4.17). The incision is then continued posteriorly close to the inferior border of the submandibular gland to avoid injuring the marginal mandibular branch of the facial nerve.

The marginal nerve runs within the thickness of the submandibular gland fascia; see Fig. 2.17. Identifying it is usually tedious and unnecessary. Safe preservation of this branch of the facial nerve may be accomplished by using the facial vein as a retractor and preserver. This maneuver begins with the identification of the facial vein at the lower border of the submandibular gland (▶ Fig. 4.18). The vein is then ligated and divided. The distal ligature is left long, with a hemostat attached, so that it can be reflected superiorly over the body of the mandible (▶ Fig. 4.19). Finally, the fascia is dissected from the surface of the submandibular gland. As the fascia and the distal stump of the anterior facial vein are retracted superiorly, the marginal mandibular branch of the facial nerve is taken away from the dissection that follows.

The dissection is then continued over the anterior border of the submandibular gland. The gland is dissected

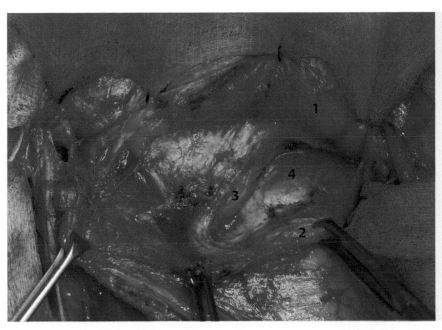

Fig. 4.17 The fascia has been incised at the upper boundary of the surgical field and retracted inferiorly along with the tissue of the submental region (right side of the neck). 1, superior skin flap; 2, fascia retracted inferiorly; 3, submandibular gland; 4, anterior belly of the digastric muscle.

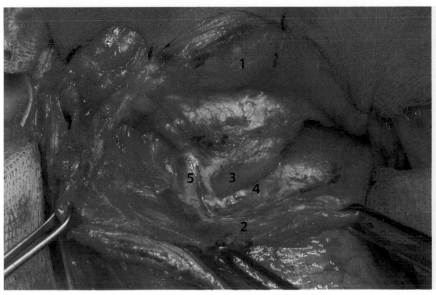

Fig. 4.18 The incision of the fascia progresses posteriorly following the inferior margin of the submandibular gland, exposing the facial vein. 1, superior skin flap; 2, fascia retracted inferiorly; 3, submandibular gland; 4, digastric muscle; 5, facial vein.

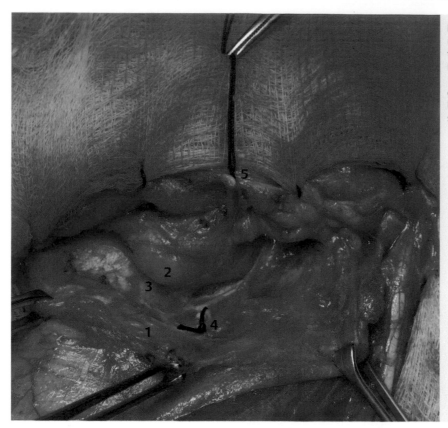

Fig. 4.19 Surgical maneuver to preserve the marginal nerve on the right side of the neck: The facial vein is ligated and divided, and the distal ligature is left long and reflected superiorly. 1, fascia retracted inferiorly; 2, submandibular gland; 3, digastric muscle; 4, facial vein (proximal ligature); 5, facial vein (distal ligature reflected superiorly).

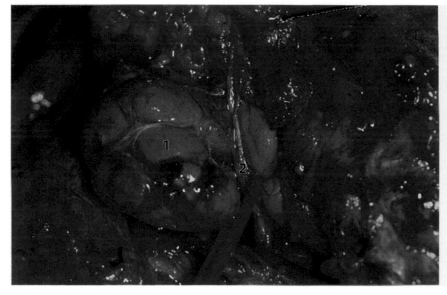

Fig. 4.20 Facial artery running superficial to the right submandibular gland. 1, submandibular gland; 2, facial artery.

posteriorly from the anterior belly of the digastric muscle, and the mylohyoid muscle is exposed. The posterior border of the mylohyoid muscle is dissected free from the submandibular gland and retracted anteriorly. The dissection continues along the superior border of the submandibular gland to identify the facial artery that may go superficial to, be embedded within, or even go posterior to the submandibular gland. The artery is ligated and divided, thus freeing the superior border of the gland. When

the facial artery goes superficial to the submandibular gland it may be dissected from the submandibular gland and preserved (▶ Fig. 4.20).

The lingual nerve must be identified by retracting the mylohyoid muscle anteriorly and the submandibular gland in a posteroinferior direction. In so doing, the traction to the submandibular ganglion, which is attached to the gland and the nerve, will bring the lingual nerve into the field (▶ Fig. 4.21). The lingual nerve can be identified

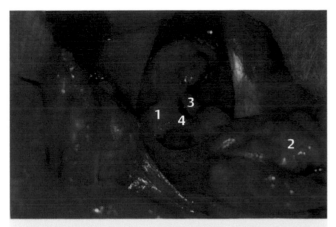

Fig. 4.21 Lingual nerve in the submandibular fossa (right side of the neck). 1, lingual nerve; 2, submandibular gland; 3, Wharton duct; 4, submandibular ganglion and accompanying vein.

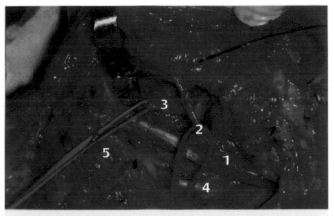

Fig. 4.22 Right submandibular fossa after removal of the submandibular gland. 1, digastric muscle; 2, facial artery; 3, lingual nerve; 4, hypoglossal nerve; 5, specimen including the submandibular gland and the lymphatic tissue from the submandibular region.

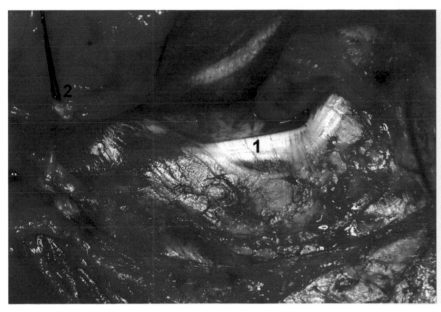

Fig. 4.23 The posterior belly of the digastric muscle leading to the forthcoming dissection (right side of the neck). 1, intermediate tendon of the digastric muscle; 2, distal ligature of the facial vein.

as a flat **V**-shaped structure in the depth of the submandibular region. The submandibular ganglion is then divided from the gland. This frees the lingual nerve, which retracts superiorly, out of the field. A vein accompanies the submandibular ganglion and should be coagulated or ligated before dividing it from the gland. The submandibular duct is identified inferior to the lingual nerve. After it has been ligated and divided, the gland is retracted inferiorly to identify the genioglossus and hyoglossus muscles. The dissection is continued inferiorly on the medial side of the submandibular gland to identify the digastric muscle and the proximal end of the facial artery. The hypoglossal nerve is identified coursing in an anterosuperior direction just above and medial to the anterior belly of the digastric muscle. The facial artery is ligated again immediately above the digastric muscle. This completely frees the submandibular gland (▶ Fig. 4.22), which is included in the specimen along with the fibrofatty tissue containing the

lymph nodes from the submandibular and submental regions (area I).

The specimen is reflected inferiorly, and the fascia over the digastric and stylohyoid muscles is incised from the midline to the tail of the parotid gland (▶ Fig. 4.23). Following the posterior belly of the digastric muscle, the stylomandibular ligament is transected (▶ Fig. 4.24).

At this level, the retromandibular vein, the posterior auricular vein, and the external jugular vein are identified. They should be ligated and divided according to their anatomical distribution. Depending on the lower extension of the tail of the parotid gland, part of the gland may also be included in the resection. This will facilitate the visualization of the upper jugular nodes (upper part of area II) as well as include in the specimen the infraparotid lymph nodes.

The digastric and stylohyoid muscles are retracted superiorly, exposing the hypoglossal nerve as well as the

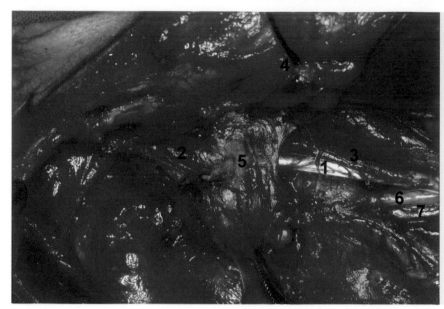

Fig. 4.24 Section of the stylomandibular ligament on the right side of the neck. 1, intermediate tendon of the digastric muscle; 2, posterior belly of the digastric muscle; 3, stylohyoid muscle; 4, distal ligature of the facial vein; 5, stylomandibular ligament; 6, hypoglossal nerve; 7, lingual vein.

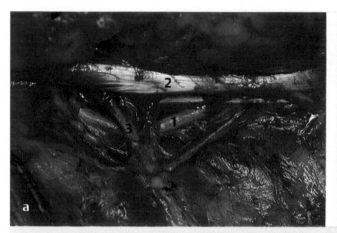

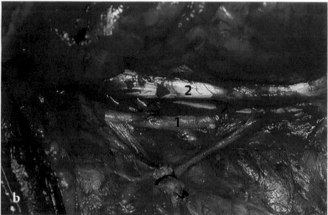

Fig. 4.25 Hypoglossal nerve in the right submandibular fossa. (a) The hypoglossal nerve is identified underneath the intermediate tendon of the digastric muscle. A lingual vein can be seen crossing superficial to the nerve. (b) The lingual vein has been ligated and the nerve is separated from the lymphatic tissue in the submandibular triangle. 1, hypoglossal nerve; 2, intermediate tendon of the digastric muscle; 3, lingual vein crossing the hypoglossal nerve.

lingual veins that follow and cross the nerve in this area (▶ Fig. 4.25). The lingual veins should be carefully ligated because they may be a source of troublesome bleeding. When bleeding occurs in this area, bipolar coagulation may be used instead of clamps and ligatures to avoid injury to the hypoglossal nerve.

The dissected tissue is finally pulled inferiorly and dissected free from the subdigastric and upper jugular spaces. At this moment, the specimen includes the submandibular and submental lymph nodes (area I), the uppermost jugular nodes (upper part of area II), and (optionally) the submandibular gland.

4.8 Dissection of the Spinal Accessory Nerve

The dissection of the spinal accessory nerve is one of the few steps of the operation that we usually perform using scissors instead of scalpel. To approach this area the sternocleidomastoid muscle is retracted posteriorly, and the posterior belly of the digastric muscle is pulled superiorly with a smooth blade retractor (▶ Fig. 4.26). This maneuver exposes the internal jugular vein and the external carotid artery. The wet surgical sponges previously left over the

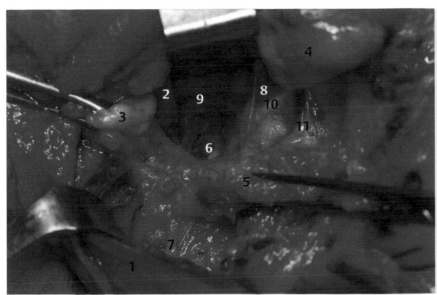

Fig. 4.26 Surgical field prepared for the dissection of the spinal accessory area on the right side of the neck. 1, sternocleidomastoid muscle; 2, digastric muscle (retracted); 3, tail of the parotid gland; 4, submandibular gland (preserved); 5, fascia dissected from the upper part of the surgical field; 6, internal jugular vein; 7, spinal accessory nerve; 8, external carotid artery; 9, occipital artery crossing the internal jugular vein; 10, hypoglossal nerve crossing the external carotid artery; 11, facial vein.

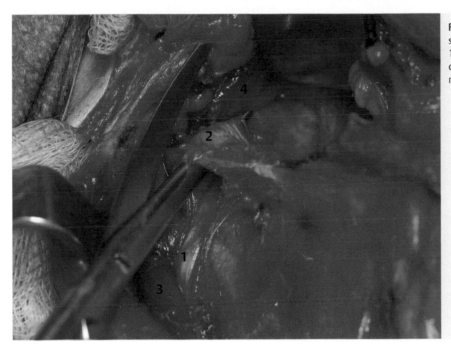

Fig. 4.27 A fascial tunnel that surrounds the spinal accessory nerve facilitates its dissection. 1, spinal accessory nerve; 2, fibrofatty tissue covering the nerve; 3, sternocleidomastoid muscle; 4, digastric muscle (retracted).

nerve at the level of its entrance in the sternocleidomastoid muscle are removed and the nerve is dissected toward the carotid sheath.

At this level the nerve runs within the "lymphatic container" of the neck, thus forcing the surgeon to cut across the fibrofatty tissue instead of following fascial planes as for the rest of the operation. This is the reason why scissors are more useful than scalpel at this stage of the operation. A fascial tunnel that surrounds the nerve enables the dissection (▶ Fig. 4.27). Consequently, the tissue overlying the nerve is divided and the nerve is completely exposed from the sternocleidomastoid muscle to the internal jugular vein (▶ Fig. 4.28a).

As the dissection approaches the internal jugular vein, the surgeon must be aware of the relationship between these two structures. Usually, the internal jugular vein lies immediately behind the proximal portion of the nerve. However, on some occasions the nerve may go behind the vein or even across it (see Fig. 2.20 and Fig. 2.21). These anatomical variations should be kept in mind to avoid unintentional damage to the internal jugular vein when following the spinal accessory nerve. The point at which the spinal accessory nerve crosses the internal jugular vein may be identified by palpating the transverse process of the atlas (▶ Fig. 4.28b).

Once the spinal accessory nerve has been completely exposed, the tissue lying superior and posterior to the nerve must be dissected from the splenius capitis and levator scapulae muscles. The tissue is pulled in an

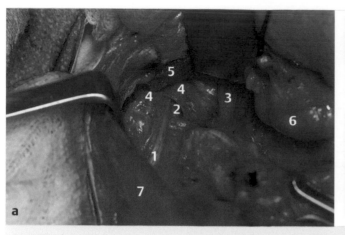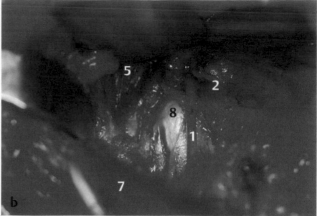

Fig. 4.28 The spinal accessory has been dissected. (a) The nerve is completely exposed in the upper part of the field on the right side of the neck. (b) Relationship between the transverse process of the atlas, the spinal accessory nerve, and the internal jugular vein. 1, spinal accessory nerve; 2, internal jugular vein; 3, external carotid artery; 4, fibrofatty tissue of the upper jugular and upper spinal accessory regions; 5, digastric muscle (retracted); 6, submandibular gland (preserved); 7, sternocleidomastoid muscle; 8, transverse process of the atlas.

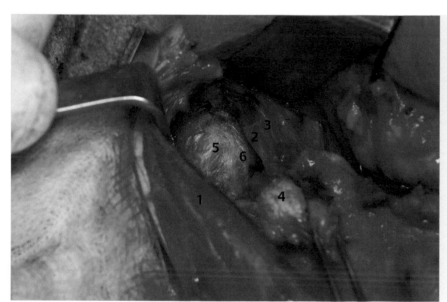

Fig. 4.29 The tissue superior and posterior to the spinal accessory nerve (area IIB) has been dissected and retracted inferiorly.
1, sternocleidomastoid muscle; 2, internal jugular vein; 3, spinal accessory nerve (displaced by the traction of the dissected tissue); 4, fibrofatty tissue retracted inferiorly; 5, splenius capitis; 6, levator scapulae muscles.

anteroinferior direction toward the spinal accessory nerve (▶ Fig. 4.29).

It must be emphasized that the lymph nodes that are now being removed are located between the spinal accessory nerve and the internal jugular vein. This region corresponds to the ill-defined boundary between area II and the upper part of area V, which constitutes one of the weak points of the artificial lymph nodal region classification. The lymph nodes in this region belong to the spinal accessory nerve lymph chain and to the upper jugular lymph chain, and no clear anatomical landmarks can be found here to separate these two lymphatic chains (▶ Fig. 4.30). Thus, the surgeon must be especially careful during this step of the operation to avoid missing potentially metastatic lymph nodes behind when performing a selective neck dissection.

The occipital and sternocleidomastoid arteries are often found at this step of the operation (▶ Fig. 4.26). When seen, they must be ligated and divided. However, most of the time they are inadvertently sectioned during the removal of the lymphatic tissue in this area. If this happens it is usually easier to cauterize them instead of trying to place clamps and ligatures.

Once the dissected tissue reaches the level of the spinal accessory nerve it must be passed underneath the nerve to be removed in continuity with the main part of the specimen. Osvaldo Suárez referred to this step of the operation as "the spinal accessory maneuver" (▶ Fig. 4.31). After this maneuver has been completed, the specimen includes the fibrofatty tissue coming from the spinal accessory nerve area along with the tissue removed from the submandibular triangle (area I) and upper jugular region (▶ Fig. 4.32).

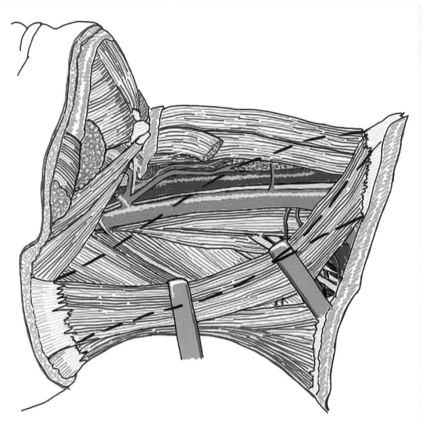

Fig. 4.30 Posterior retraction of the sternocleidomastoid muscle distorts the theoretic limits between level II and the upper part of level V on an area without significant anatomic landmarks. The dotted lines show the original position of the muscle. Depending on the retraction, the limit between the two levels may vary.

Before moving to the next step of the operation, a final cut is made in this area that will help further dissection. Keeping the sternocleidomastoid muscle retracted posteriorly, a number-10 scalpel blade is used to make an incision into the tissue located below the entrance of the spinal accessory nerve into the sternocleidomastoid muscle. This cut is made just anterior to the sternocleidomastoid muscle and goes down to the level of Erb's point following the medial border of the sternocleidomastoid muscle (▶ Fig. 4.33). The underlying levator scapulae muscle is identified and the tissue is slightly dissected forward and medially over its fascia. The rest of the dissection in this area will be completed later.

Again, wet surgical sponges are left around the spinal accessory nerve over the splenius capitis and levator scapulae muscles, and the dissection is taken to the supraclavicular fossa.

4.9 Dissection of the Posterior Triangle of the Neck

The supraclavicular fossa constitutes the lower part of area V. The need to include this area in the dissection has been one of the most controversial issues concerning functional and selective neck dissection. We remind the reader that this controversy is beyond the scope of this book. Neither are we discussing the indications for the inclusion of this region in the dissection, nor are we suggesting that this should be considered an unavoidable part of functional neck dissection for every single head-and-neck tumor. As should be clear to those reaching this point of reading, *functional* is not a surgical technique, but a concept, and the description of a complete approach should mention the removal of all nodal groups in the neck.

A comprehensive exposure of the supraclavicular area has usually been performed posterior to the sternocleidomastoid muscle, by gentle anterior retraction of the muscle. The dissection begins with the removal of the fascia that still covers the posterior border of the sternocleidomastoid muscle (▶ Fig. 4.34). It must be remembered that the fascia was dissected off the muscle up to its posterior border in a previous step of the operation (see section "Dissection of the Sternocleidomastoid Muscle"). The wet surgical sponges left between the anteromedial aspect of the muscle and the dissected fascia are used as a reference to complete the fascial isolation of the sternocleidomastoid muscle. Once completed, this maneuver results in a total release of the muscle from its surrounding fascia (▶ Fig. 4.35).

The loose fibrofatty tissue of the supraclavicular fossa and the absence of well-defined dissection planes within this area make knife dissection ineffective here. Thus, for this step of the operation, scissors and blunt dissection are preferred.

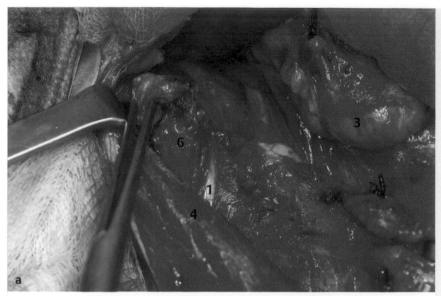

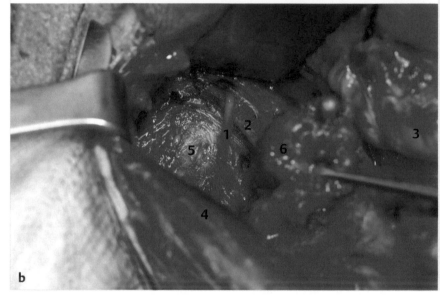

Fig. 4.31 Spinal accessory maneuver on the right side of the neck. (a) The nerve is exposed between the sternocleidomastoid muscle and the internal jugular vein. (b) The fibrofatty tissue lying posterior and superior to the nerve is passed beneath the nerve. 1, spinal accessory nerve; 2, internal jugular vein; 3, submandibular gland (preserved); 4, sternocleidomastoid muscle; 5, splenius capitis and levator scapulae muscles; 6, specimen from the upper spinal accessory and posterosuperior jugular area.

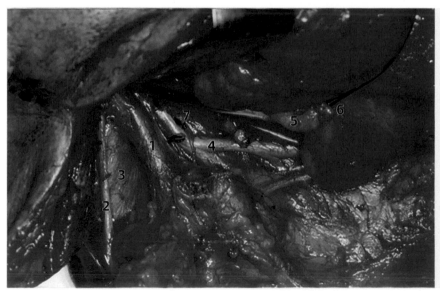

Fig. 4.32 Anterior view of the surgical field after dissection of the upper cervical regions on the right side of the neck. 1, internal jugular vein; 2, spinal accessory nerve; 3, levator scapulae muscle; 4, hypoglossal nerve; 5, submandibular gland; 6, distal ligature of the facial vein; 7, divided lingual veins.

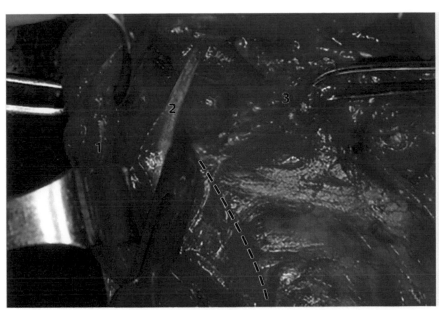

Fig. 4.33 The spinal accessory maneuver has been completed. A final cut is made anterior to the sternocleidomastoid muscle (dashed line), between the spinal accessory nerve and the level of Erb's point (right side of the neck).
1, sternocleidomastoid muscle retracted posteriorly; 2, spinal accessory nerve; 3, specimen from the upper jugular and spinal accessory area.

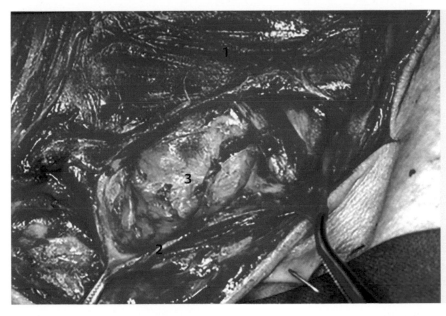

Fig. 4.34 Dissection of the remaining fascia of the sternocleidomastoid muscle at the supraclavicular fossa (right side of the neck).
1, sternocleidomastoid muscle; 2, fascia retracted laterally; 3, fibrofatty tissue of the supraclavicular fossa.

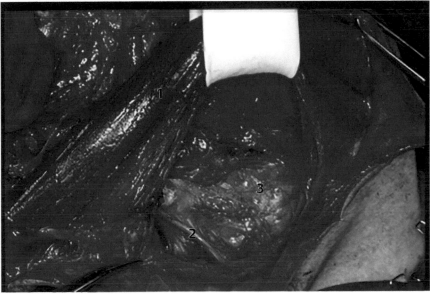

Fig. 4.35 The sternocleidomastoid muscle is completely released from its surrounding fascia and is pulled medially to facilitate the dissection of the supraclavicular fossa (right side of the neck). 1, sternocleidomastoid muscle retracted medially; 2, supraclavicular branch of the cervical plexus; 3, fibrofatty tissue of the supraclavicular fossa.

4

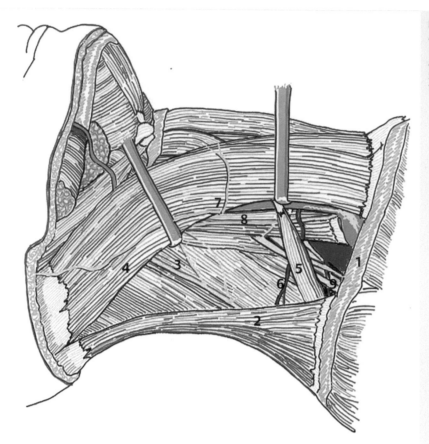

Fig. 4.36 Boundaries of the dissection and anatomic landmarks in the posterior triangle. 1, clavicle; 2, trapezius muscle; 3, spinal accessory nerve; 4, sternocleidomastoid muscle; 5, omohyoid muscle; 6, transverse cervical artery; 7, Erb's point; 8, phrenic nerve; 9, brachial plexus.

Some anatomical landmarks define the boundaries of the surgical field in the posterior triangle (▶ Fig. 4.36). The inferior limit is located at the level of the clavicle. The posterior margin is clearly marked by the anterior edge of the trapezius muscle, and the upper boundary is defined by the exit of the spinal accessory nerve toward the trapezius muscle. The transverse cervical vessels and the omohyoid muscle constitute important anatomical landmarks within this area.

For a classic posterior approach, the sternocleidomastoid muscle is retracted anteriorly, and the external jugular vein is divided and ligated low in the neck if this was not done at a previous stage of the operation. The dissection then proceeds from the anterior border of the trapezius muscle in a medial direction including the lymphatic contents of the supraclavicular fossa. The upper margin of this area presents the greatest risk of damage to the spinal accessory nerve. The spinal accessory nerve leaves the sternocleidomastoid muscle deep to Erb's point and descends obliquely downward and backward toward the trapezius muscle. The position of the patient's head, along with the traction exerted by the surgeon during the dissection may displace the nerve from its original course, creating a slight anterior curvature where the nerve may be inadvertently damaged. Displacement of the nerve is due to its connections with the second, third, and fourth cervical nerves. During the dissection of this region

several supraclavicular branches of the cervical plexus may be found. They follow a similar course but are located superficially and inferiorly to the spinal accessory nerve (▶ Fig. 4.37). Although the difference between the eleventh nerve and the supraclavicular branches is easily noticed, the novice surgeon may sometimes find this to be difficult.

The omohyoid muscle is then identified, and its fascia is dissected off the muscle to be removed with the contents of the posterior triangle. The muscle may be transected at this moment if this will be required for the removal of the primary tumor; otherwise it is preserved and retracted inferiorly with a smooth blade retractor. The transverse cervical vessels are identified deep to the omohyoid muscle (▶ Fig. 4.38). Usually they are easily dissected free from the surrounding fibrofatty tissue, displaced inferiorly, and preserved. However, the numerous variations in the branches and the exact manner of branching of the thyrocervical trunk restrain the systematization of this step (▶ Fig. 4.39).

The deep layer of the cervical fascia over the levator scapulae and scalene muscles is now visible (▶ Fig. 4.38). The brachial plexus is easily identified as it appears between the anterior and middle scalene. Staying superficial to the scalene fascia prevents injuring the brachial plexus and the phrenic nerve (▶ Fig. 4.40).

The dissection is continued medially until it reaches the level of the anterior border of the sternocleidomastoid

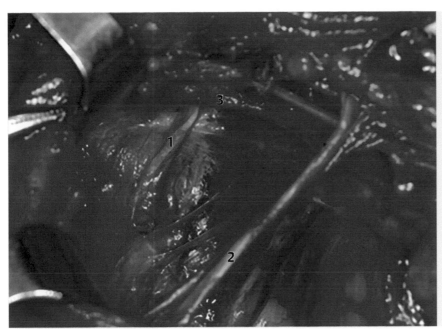

Fig. 4.37 The spinal accessory nerve crossing the posterior triangle of the neck on the right side. Note the supraclavicular branch of the cervical plexus following a similar course, but more superficially and more inferiorly. 1, spinal accessory nerve; 2, supraclavicular branch of the cervical plexus; 3, sternocleidomastoid muscle (posterior border).

4

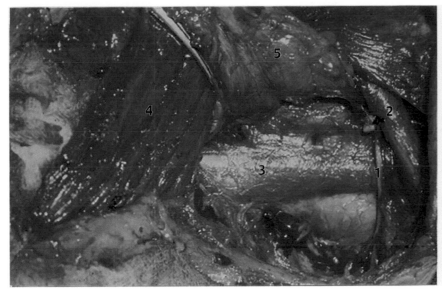

Fig. 4.38 Dissection of the right supraclavicular fossa. 1, transverse cervical artery; 2, omohyoid muscle; 3, anterior scalene muscle; 4, sternocleidomastoid muscle; 5, specimen from the supraclavicular fossa.

muscle. The muscle is then pulled laterally with retractors and the contents of the supraclavicular fossa are passed underneath to meet the tissue previously dissected from the upper half of the neck. The sternocleidomastoid muscle is then retracted posteriorly, and the dissection continues anterior to the muscle toward the carotid sheath.

For those who prefer to perform the whole operation anterior to the sternocleidomastoid muscle, the removal of the tissue from the supraclavicular area is also possible as long as the muscle is strongly retracted posteriorly and the skin incision has been properly designed along the posterior border of the sternocleidomastoid muscle.

4.10 Dissection of the Deep Cervical Muscles

If the previous steps have been properly performed, we will now have two main blocks of the dissection. The upper part includes the submandibular and submental triangles (area I), as well as the upper jugular and spinal accessory regions (upper part of areas II and V). The lower block includes the supraclavicular fossa (remaining part of area V). A small bridge of tissue still separates these two blocks and connects the specimen to the deep cervical muscles (▶ Fig. 4.41). This bridge usually goes from just below the entrance of the spinal accessory nerve into the

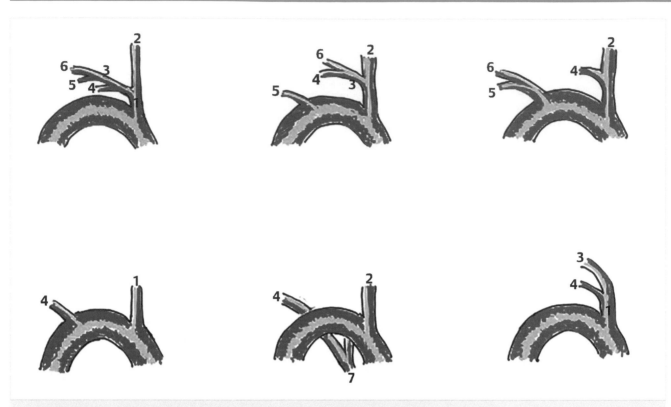

Fig. 4.39 Variations in the branches of the thyrocervical trunk. 1, thyrocervical trunk; 2, inferior thyroid artery; 3, transverse cervical artery; 4, superficial cervical artery; 5, descending scapular artery; 6, suprascapular artery; 7, internal thoracic artery.

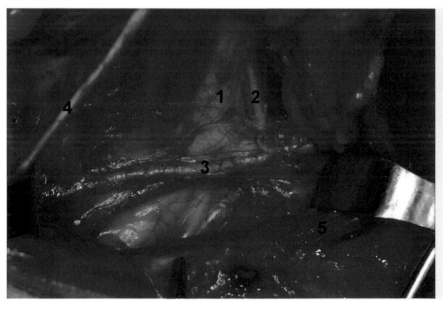

Fig. 4.40 Anterior view of the anatomic landmarks on the right supraclavicular fossa. 1, brachial plexus; 2, phrenic nerve; 3, transverse cervical artery; 4, supraclavicular branch of the cervical plexus; 5, omohyoid muscle retracted inferomedially.

sternocleidomastoid muscle to a level just below Erb's point.

Using a scalpel, this bridge is transected and the fascia of the levator scapulae muscle is identified. This maneuver creates a single block that must be dissected free from the deep muscles toward the carotid sheath (▶ Fig. 4.42). The dissection that follows will be performed using sharp dissection. Thus, the specimen is grasped with forceps, and adequate traction is applied.

As the dissection proceeds medially, several branches of the cervical plexus are found. A thorough knowledge of neck anatomy is essential to combine oncological radicalism with functional surgery. As already mentioned, to achieve optimal shoulder function, the deep branches from the second, third, and fourth cervical nerves that may anastomose with the spinal accessory nerve should be preserved (▶ Fig. 4.43). In the same manner, the contribution to the phrenic nerve from the third, fourth, and

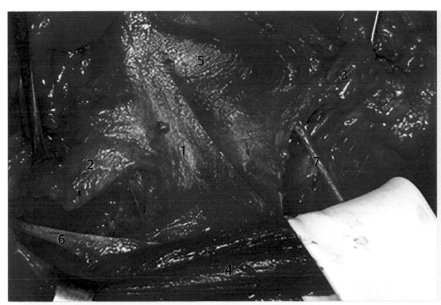

Fig. 4.41 Lateral view of the bridge of tissue between the upper and the lower parts of the specimen on a right functional neck dissection. 1, bridge of tissue between the upper and lower parts of the specimen; 2, upper part of the specimen (submandibular, upper jugular, and upper spinal accessory regions); 3, lower part of the specimen (supraclavicular area); 4, sternocleidomastoid muscle retracted laterally; 5, internal jugular vein; 6, spinal accessory nerve; 7, supraclavicular branch of the cervical plexus.

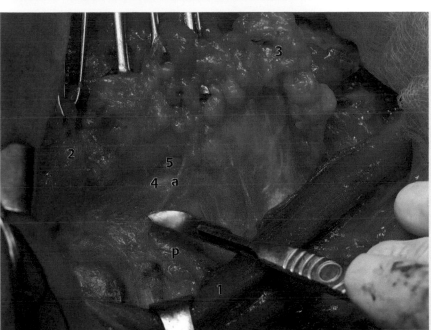

Fig. 4.42 The whole specimen is now anterior to the sternocleidomastoid muscle. Note the anterior (a) and posterior (p) branch of the cervical plexus. The anterior branches must be sectioned to continue the dissection toward the carotid sheath (right side of the neck). 1, sternocleidomastoid muscle; 2, upper part of the specimen (submandibular, upper jugular, and upper spinal accessory areas); 3, lower part of the specimen (supraclavicular fossa); 4, carotid artery; 5, internal jugular vein.

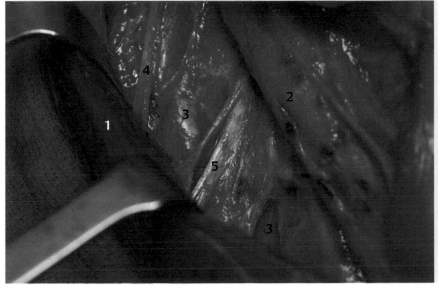

Fig. 4.43 Lateral view of the deep branches of the cervical plexus that have been preserved on the right side of the neck. 1, sternocleidomastoid muscle; 2, carotid artery; 3, deep cervical muscles; 4, spinal accessory nerve; 5, deep branches of the cervical plexus.

4

fifth cervical nerves should also be preserved. This is best achieved by keeping the dissection superficial to the scalene fascia, where the branches of the cervical plexus usually lie. On the other hand, the superficial or anterior cutaneous branches of the cervical plexus will be transected as the dissection approaches the carotid sheath.

The dissection of the deep cervical muscles must be stopped as soon as the carotid sheath is exposed. Continuing the dissection posterior to the carotid sheath carries a high risk of damage to the sympathetic trunk (▶ Fig. 4.44).

4.11 Dissection of the Carotid Sheath

The carotid sheath is a fascial envelope surrounding the internal jugular vein, common carotid artery, and vagus nerve; see Fig. 2.3. It is interposed between the three layers of the cervical fascia. The carotid sheath must be included in the resection, preserving its neurovascular contents.

This part of the dissection needs a new number-10 knife blade and adequate tension. The surgical specimen is grasped with hemostats and retracted medially by the assistant, while the surgeon uses one hand with a gauze pad to pull laterally over the deep cervical muscles. This allows a complete exposure of the carotid sheath along the entire length of the surgical field. To avoid injuring important neurovascular structures, during the next minutes all movements should be precise and gentle. This includes all activity from the assistants, scrub nurse, and circulating personnel in the operating room.

An incision is made with the scalpel over the vagus nerve along the entire length of the carotid sheath (▶ Fig. 4.45). The nerve can be easily identified between the internal jugular vein and the carotid artery

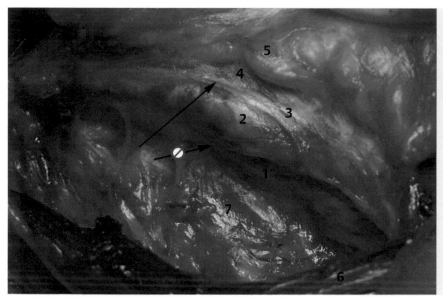

Fig. 4.44 The dissection should be carried out in a direction anterior to the carotid artery *(arrows)*, avoiding damage to the sympathetic trunk, which is located posterior to the artery. 1, sympathetic trunk; 2, carotid artery; 3, vagus nerve; 4, internal jugular vein; 5, specimen; 6, sternocleidomastoid muscle; 7, deep cervical muscles.

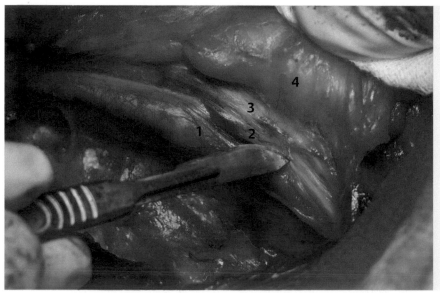

Fig. 4.45 The carotid sheath should be opened by cutting over the vagus nerve. 1, carotid artery; 2, vagus nerve; 3, internal jugular vein; 4, specimen.

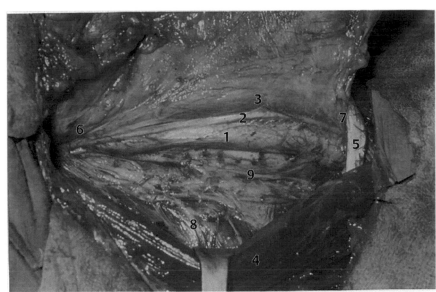

Fig. 4.46 Dissection of the carotid sheath on the right side of the neck. 1, carotid artery; 2, vagus nerve; 3, internal jugular vein; 4, sternocleidomastoid muscle; 5, omohyoid muscle; 6, upper fold of the internal jugular vein; 7, inferior fold of the internal jugular vein; 8, deep branches of the cervical plexus; 9, phrenic nerve.

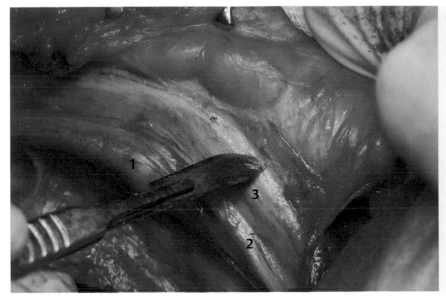

Fig. 4.47 Dissection of the carotid sheath on the right side of the neck. 1, carotid artery; 2, vagus nerve; 3, internal jugular vein.

(▶ Fig. 4.46). The dissection then continues, removing the fascia from the internal jugular vein. This is achieved by continuously passing the knife blade along the wall of the internal jugular vein up and down along its entire length (▶ Fig. 4.47). The scalpel must be moved obliquely with respect to the vein, with the blade pointing away from the vein wall. When this is properly done and the traction exerted on the tissue is adequate, this maneuver is extremely safe and effective. The fascia can be seen coming apart from the vein after each pass of the knife blade, until the internal jugular vein is completely released from its fascial covering (▶ Fig. 4.48).

The facial, lingual, and thyroid veins appear as the dissection approaches the medial wall of the internal jugular vein (▶ Fig. 4.49). They should be clearly identified, ligated, and divided to complete the isolation of the internal jugular vein. Other smaller branches as well as some vasa vasorum

often found during the dissection of the internal jugular vein can be cauterized, taking care not to use the cautery too close to the venous wall to avoid troublesome perforations that will require further repair. Bipolar cautery may be helpful at this stage of the operation.

The dissection of the carotid sheath has two danger points. One at each end—upper and lower—of the dissection (▶ Fig. 4.46). At these two points the traction exerted to facilitate the dissection of the fascial envelope produces a folding of the wall of the internal jugular vein that can be easily sectioned at the touch of the scalpel blade. We refer to these two points as the *initial folds*, and they should be freed before further dissection of the internal jugular vein is attempted. The surgeon must be extremely cautious to avoid injuring the vein at these points.

Lower in the neck, the terminal portion of the thoracic duct on the left side (▶ Fig. 4.50) and the right lymphatic

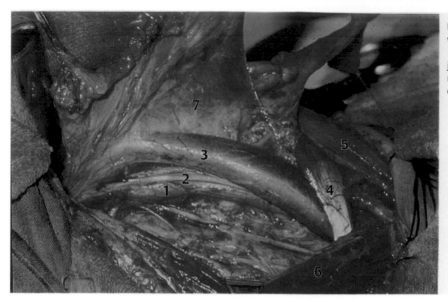

Fig. 4.48 Dissection of the internal jugular vein within the carotid sheath (right side of the neck). 1, carotid artery; 2, vagus nerve; 3, internal jugular vein; 4, omohyoid muscle; 5, sternohyoid muscle; 6, sternocleidomastoid muscle; 7, fascia of the carotid sheath.

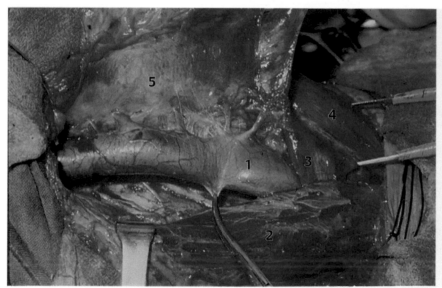

Fig. 4.49 Lateral view of the veins draining into the medial face of the right internal jugular vein. 1, internal jugular vein; 2, sternocleidomastoid muscle; 3, omohyoid muscle; 4, sternohyoid muscle; 5, fascia of the carotid sheath.

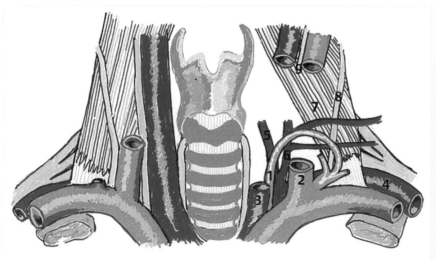

Fig. 4.50 Cervical course of the thoracic duct on the left side of the neck. 1, thoracic duct; 2, internal jugular vein; 3, carotid artery; 4, subclavian artery; 5, vertebral artery; 6, thyrocervical trunk; 7, anterior scalene muscle; 8, phrenic nerve; 9, vagus nerve.

duct, when present, are also within the boundaries of the dissection and must be preserved. They are difficult to identify because of their variable anatomy and, more often than desired, can only be found after being injured, which is especially likely given their very thin wall that easily breaks under normal dissection maneuvers. The surgeon must be aware that postoperative leakage in patients with functional neck dissection is much more difficult to solve than in patients with radical neck dissection because of the preservation of the sternocleidomastoid muscle. The pressure maneuvers that usually control chylous leaks in patients with radical neck dissection are less effective when the muscle remains in place. Thus, intraoperative recognition of the problem and appropriate management at the time of operation are essential for a successful outcome. Once injured, the thoracic duct must be surrounded by muscle, fascia, or adipose tissue before being sutured. More details about the management of the thoracic duct can be found in Chapter 5.

Once the branches of the internal jugular vein are divided and the vein is completely released from its covering fascia, the dissection continues medially over the carotid artery to reach the strap muscles. The traction applied to the specimen usually displaces the superior thyroid artery anteriorly, and it comes into the plane of dissection. Its identification when reaching to the carotid bifurcation prevents accidental damage to the artery (▶ Fig. 4.51).

The specimen is finally completely separated from the great vessels and remains attached only to the strap muscles. The dissection of the strap muscles will complete the release of the neck dissection specimen. However, when the strap muscles are to be removed with the primary tumor, an en bloc resection may be performed by leaving the specimen pedicled over the strap muscles in order to resect the primary tumor in-continuity with the neck dissection specimen.

The specimen of a functional neck dissection has been classically compared to a butterfly, with two wings and a body. The body is formed by the carotid sheath. One wing covers the strap muscles and the other wing includes the lateral contents of the dissection.

4.12 Dissection of the Strap Muscles

Although this is described as the last step of the operation, it may be performed in a different order according to the needs of the surgery and the location of the primary tumor. Conversely to the rest of the procedure, the dissection at this level is performed from medial to lateral. Thus, a midline cut is made in the superficial layer of the cervical fascia from the upper border of the surgical field to the sternal notch (▶ Fig. 4.52).

The fascia is then dissected from the underlying strap muscles. The dissection starts at the upper part of the surgical field and continues in a lateral and inferior direction. The anterior jugular vein is ligated and divided at its origin (at the level of the hyoid bone) and at the lower boundary of the dissection. The sternohyoid and omohyoid muscles are completely freed from their fascial covering (▶ Fig. 4.53). The common facial vein, the anterior jugular vein, and a variable vein communicating the superficial and deep venous systems of the neck (Kocher's vein) are usually ligated and divided before the specimen is completely released from the strap muscles.

4.13 Closure of the Wound

▶ Fig. 4.54 and ▶ Fig. 4.55 show the appearance of the neck after functional neck dissection has been completed. Once again, we would like to emphasize that it is not the

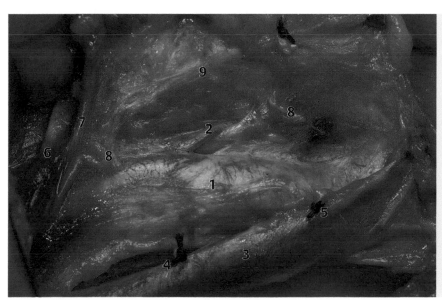

Fig. 4.51 Identification of the superior thyroid artery before finishing the dissection of the carotid sheath (right side of the neck). 1, carotid bifurcation; 2, superior thyroid artery; 3, internal jugular vein; 4, thyro-linguo-facial vein (ligated); 5, middle thyroid vein (ligated); 6, digastric and stylohyoid muscles; 7, hypoglossal nerve; 8, superior root of ansa cervicalis (divided); 9, specimen.

4

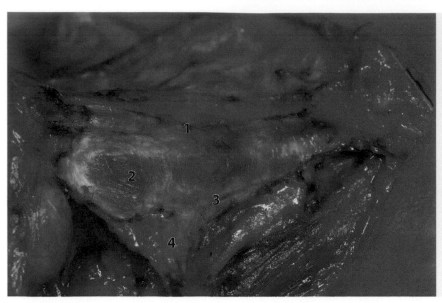

Fig. 4.52 The dissection of the strap muscles starts by performing a midline incision in the cervical fascia and reflecting the specimen laterally. 1, midline; 2, sternohyoid muscle; 3, anterior jugular vein; 4, specimen reflected laterally.

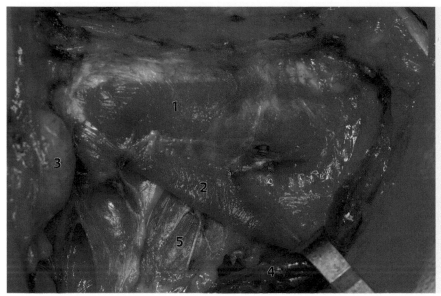

Fig. 4.53 The dissection of the strap muscles has already finished. 1, sternohyoid muscle; 2, omohyoid muscle; 3, submandibular gland; 4, sternocleidomastoid muscle; 5, final attachment of the specimen.

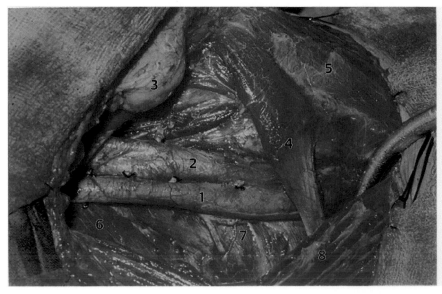

Fig. 4.54 The neck after a right functional neck dissection. 1, internal jugular vein; 2, carotid artery; 3, submandibular gland; 4, omohyoid muscle; 5, sternohyoid muscle; 6, levator scapulae muscle; 7, anterior scalene muscle; 8, sternocleidomastoid muscle.

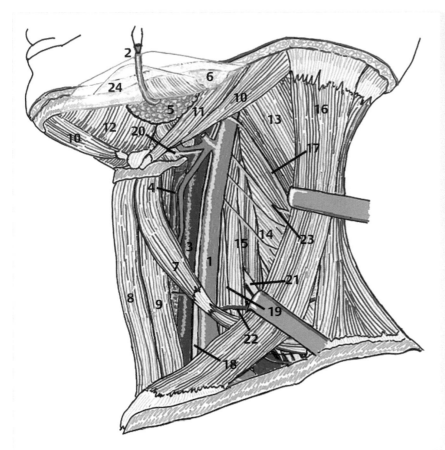

Fig. 4.55 The neck after functional neck dissection. 1, internal jugular vein; 2, distal stump of the facial vein; 3, common carotid artery; 4, superior thyroid artery; 5, submandibular gland; 6, parotid gland; 7, omohyoid muscle; 8, sternohyoid muscle; 9, sternothyroid muscle; 10, digastric muscle; 11, stylohyoid muscle; 12, mylohyoid muscle; 13, splenius capitis muscle; 14, levator scapulae muscle; 15, scalene muscles; 16, sternocleidomastoid muscle; 17, spinal accessory nerve; 18, vagus nerve; 19, phrenic nerve; 20, hypoglossal nerve; 21, brachial plexus; 22, transverse cervical artery; 23, deep branches of the cervical plexus; 24, marginal branch of the facial nerve.

4

preservation of anatomical structures that makes functional neck dissection different from radical neck dissection, but the approach to the neck through fascial planes.

The neck is carefully inspected for bleeding points and surgical sponges. Careful hemostasis is time consuming but rewarding. The entire field is thoroughly irrigated with warm saline. Finally, the skin is closed in two layers over a large suction catheter. The platysma is sutured with absorbable buried sutures, and the skin with skin clips. A moderately tight dressing is applied with special attention to the supraclavicular fossa because this is the area where most serohematomas develop.

4.14 Dissection of the Central Compartment

The prelaryngeal, pretracheal, and paratracheal lymph nodes constitute the central lymphatic compartment of the neck (area VI). Lymph nodes in this area are mainly located in the tracheoesophageal groove and around the recurrent laryngeal nerves. For some tumor locations, the central compartment must be included in the dissection. This is the case of tumors of the thyroid gland, subglottic lesions, and some hypopharyngeal cancers. In some cases, it is also important to remove the lymph nodes in the

anterior superior mediastinum along with the dissection of the central compartment.

The lateral boundaries of this region are the common carotid arteries. The inferior boundary is the brachiocephalic trunk on the right side and a similar level on the left side. The superior anatomic boundary is the hyoid bone. However, the central compartment dissection is rarely carried out further up than the level of the cricoid cartilage, especially when dealing with a thyroid cancer, as the risk of metastases above this level is scarce and the dissection is so complex when performed through a thyroidectomy incision.

The approach starts with the dissection of the ipsilateral thyroid lobe. When treating hypopharyngeal or subglottic cancers, the thyroid lobe may be removed en bloc with the larynx. The recurrent laryngeal nerve and both parathyroid glands should be identified during thyroidectomy. Due to the different anatomy of the recurrent laryngeal nerve, the technique of the central compartment dissection differs at each side.

On the *right side*, the nerve crosses the central compartment obliquely, and divides it into two triangles (► Fig. 4.56). The first step consists of following the nerve from up to down, from its entry in the larynx to the inferior limit of the dissection (► Fig. 4.57). The branches of the inferior thyroid artery to the inferior parathyroid

4

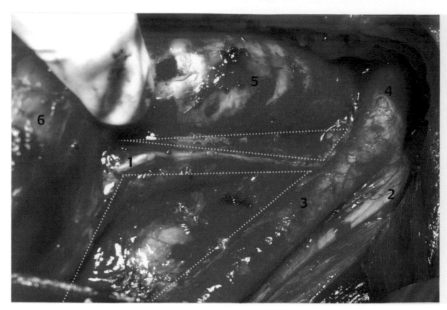

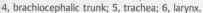

Fig. 4.56 The recurrent laryngeal nerve divides the right central compartment into two triangles. 1, recurrent laryngeal nerve entering the larynx; 2, recurrent laryngeal nerve emerging from vagus nerve; 3, common carotid artery; 4, brachiocephalic trunk; 5, trachea; 6, larynx.

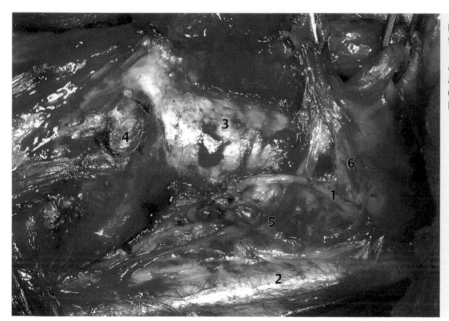

Fig. 4.57 Recurrent laryngeal nerve dissected all the way along the right central compartment. 1, recurrent laryngeal nerve; 2, common carotid artery; 3, trachea; 4, larynx; 5, specimen superior and lateral to the recurrent laryngeal nerve; 6, specimen inferior and medial to the recurrent laryngeal nerve.

gland cross the course of the nerve, which makes the correct dissection difficult; thus, these branches are usually coagulated and the gland reimplanted. Once the nerve is completely exposed, the adipose tissue in the inferior triangle of the central compartment (between the nerve laterally, the brachiocephalic trunk inferiorly, and the trachea and esophagus medially) may be removed. Next, the inferior thyroid artery is identified laterally, as it enters the compartment behind the common carotid artery. The inferior thyroid artery is then carefully followed to the superior parathyroid gland to preserve its vascularization. The inferior thyroid artery divides the superior part of the central compartment in two new triangles (▶ Fig. 4.58): the first lies between the nerve, the inferior thyroid artery, and the common carotid artery. The second is located between

the inferior thyroid artery, the common carotid artery, and the upper limit of the dissection. The adipose tissue of each triangle may be removed, with attention to preserve the recurrent laryngeal nerve and the vascular supply to the superior parathyroid gland.

The dissection on the *left side* is much easier, as the nerve runs against the tracheo-esophageal groove (▶ Fig. 4.59). Thus, after following the nerve inferiorly, all the tissue of the compartment may be reflected laterally. The inferior thyroid artery is identified laterally and its branches to the parathyroid glands followed and preserved. The vascularization of the inferior parathyroid gland is more difficult to preserve and, if needed, the gland may be removed and reimplanted. Finally, the adipose and lymphatic tissue is completely removed.

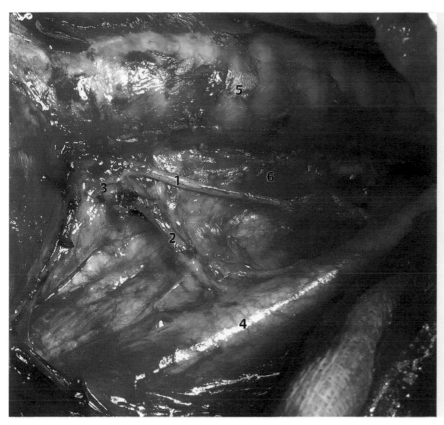

Fig. 4.58 The right central compartment after dissection. 1, recurrent laryngeal nerve; 2, inferior thyroid artery; 3, superior parathyroid gland; 4, common carotid artery; 5, trachea; 6, esophagus.

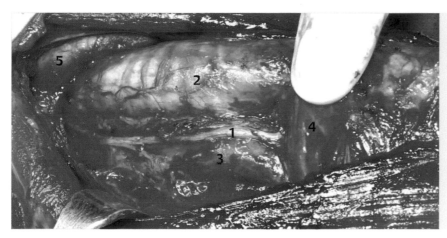

Fig. 4.59 The left recurrent laryngeal nerve crossing the central compartment. 1, recurrent laryngeal nerve; 2, trachea; 3, esophagus; 4, larynx; 5, brachiocephalic trunk.

When the primary tumor requires the removal of the ipsilateral hemilarynx, the dissection is much easier since the recurrent laryngeal nerve can be sacrificed. However, adequate management of the parathyroid glands is extremely important in all cases. Efforts should be made to preserve at least the superior parathyroid glands properly vascularized, and to reimplant in the sternocleidomastoid muscle the inferior parathyroid glands if needed. We recommend to confirm on frozen sections that it is parathyroid tissue, and not potential metastases, before reimplanting any tissue from the neck dissection area.

5 Hints and Pitfalls

5.1 Knife Dissection and the Functional Approach

The principle of fascial dissection is more easily achieved when the surgeon uses the cold knife through fascial planes. For most steps of the operation the scalpel is the best surgical tool, whereas for others the scissors are preferred. Elevation of the skin flaps and dissection of the sternocleidomastoid muscle, submandibular fossa, deep cervical muscles, carotid sheath, and strap muscles are best performed using knife dissection. On the other hand, dissection of the area around the spinal accessory nerve, posterior triangle, and paratracheal space is more easily accomplished with the scissors. The main difference between these two groups is the type of tissue that is being dissected. Knife dissection requires firm tissue like muscle or vessels (▶ Fig. 5.1), whereas fibrofatty tissue is more easily dissected with the scissors (▶ Fig. 5.2).

Knife dissection requires precise handling of the knife, careful surgical technique, and adequate help from the assistants. The blade of the scalpel must be directed oblique to the tissue that is being dissected and away from the muscle or vessel whose fascia is being removed. This protects the structures, especially the veins, from being injured by the knife blade. To be appropriate, knife dissection must be carried all the way up and down the surgical field, avoiding the creation of holes along the dissected structure. The knife blade is much more efficient when cutting over tense tissue. Thus, the assistants must apply adequate tension to the surgical field to increase the effectiveness of knife dissection.

5.2 Washing the Field Regularly

Clear vision of the different structures in the surgical field is of paramount importance. Blood obscures the field and makes identification of structures more difficult. A bloodless field must be maintained throughout the operation. In addition, washing the field regularly with warm saline greatly contributes to cleaning the working area (▶ Fig. 5.3).

5.3 Raising the Flaps

The superficial layer of the cervical fascia must remain intact after the flaps have been raised. This may pose a problem to the novice surgeon, who usually finds it difficult to preserve the integrity of this fascial layer. The best way to achieve this goal is by cutting with the scalpel over the deep face of the platysma muscle. As for any other type of neck dissection, the platysma muscle is included with the skin flaps because it provides additional blood supply that protects the skin and assists in the healing process. The proper sequence for an adequate incision will be to mark the skin incision, incise the skin, cut the platysma muscle, and start raising the flap, keeping the deep face of the platysma under vision. If the muscular fibers of the platysma are seen throughout the elevation of the skin flaps (▶ Fig. 5.4), then preservation of the superficial layer of the cervical fascia is assured.

5.4 Identification of the Great Auricular Nerve

The great auricular nerve is used to identify the posterior border of the upper part of the surgical field. This branch of the cervical plexus rounds the posterior border of the sternocleidomastoid muscle from Erb's point and courses almost directly upward toward the ear lobule, where it supplies almost all the auricle, the skin over the parotid gland, and the skin over the mastoid process.

Whenever possible, the great auricular nerve should be preserved to avoid numbness of the ear. This is facilitated by incising the fascia of the sternocleidomastoid muscle right anteriorly to the nerve. This line will mark the posterior margin of the dissection (▶ Fig. 5.5).

5.5 Management of the External Jugular Vein

The external jugular vein begins in the substance of the parotid gland. It is most often formed by the union of the retromandibular (posterior facial) and the posterior auricular veins. It runs vertically downward across the superficial surface of the sternocleidomastoid muscle to pierce the fascia of the posterior triangle of the neck just above the clavicle. The external jugular vein terminates in the subclavian or in the internal jugular vein after receiving several tributaries throughout its cervical course; see Fig. 2.12.

During functional neck dissection, the external jugular vein is found at different stages of the operation and should be ligated and divided at different levels. On a complete functional neck dissection, there are three places where the external jugular vein must be ligated and divided; see ▶ Fig. 5.6 and Fig. 4.10. From up to down, the vein must be transected: (1) at the tail of the parotid gland during the dissection of the upper part of the surgical field; (2) at the level of the posterior border of the sternocleidomastoid muscle during the dissection of the muscle; and (3) within the fibrofatty tissue of the supraclavicular fossa while dissecting the posterior triangle of the neck.

During the ligature of the external jugular vein and other large veins in the neck, special attention should be

5

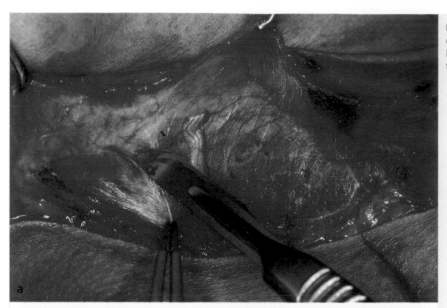

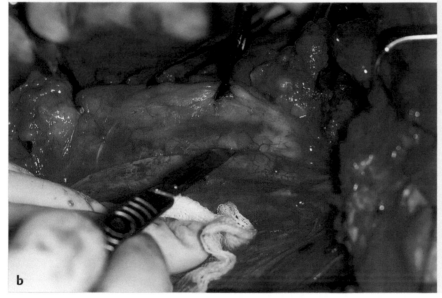

Fig. 5.1 The knife is preferred for the dissection of firm tissue like muscle (**a**) or vessels (**b**). Safe knife dissection requires placing the tissue under traction, as seen in the photos.

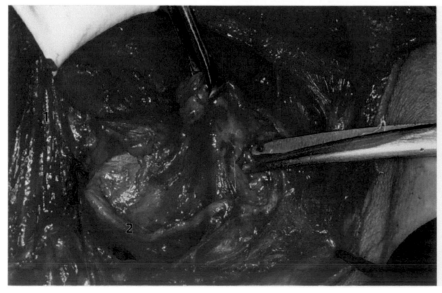

Fig. 5.2 Fibrofatty tissue is best dissected with the scissors. An example of the dissection of the supraclavicular fossa on the right side of the neck. 1, sternocleidomastoid muscle retracted medially; 2, supraclavicular nerve.

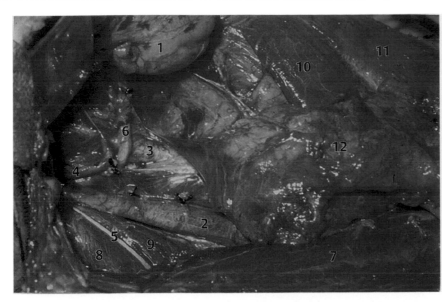

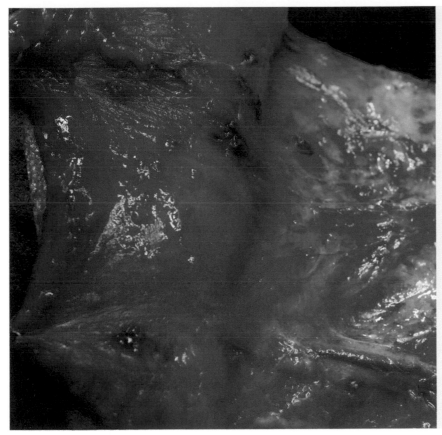

Fig. 5.3 Regularly washing the field allows better visualization of the anatomical structures. 1, submandibular gland; 2, internal jugular vein; 3, carotid artery; 4, lingual veins; 5, spinal accessory nerve; 6, hypoglossal nerve; 7, sternocleidomastoid muscle; 8, splenius capitis muscle; 9, levator scapulae muscle; 10, omohyoid muscle; 11, sternohyoid muscle; 12, neck dissection specimen.

Fig. 5.4 Fibers of the platysma muscle after elevation of the skin flaps.

5

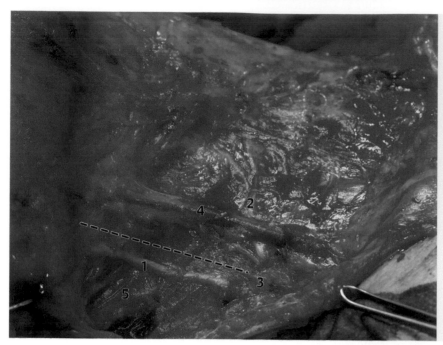

Fig. 5.5 Identification and preservation of the great auricular nerve on the right side of the neck. The great auricular nerve crosses the external face of the sternocleidomastoid muscle from Erb's point toward the ear lobule. The fascia over the sternocleidomastoid muscle is incised anterior to the great auricular nerve in order to preserve innervation of the ear lobule (dashed line). 1, great auricular nerve; 2, transverse cervical branch of the cervical plexus; 3, Erb's point; 4, external jugular vein; 5, sternocleidomastoid muscle.

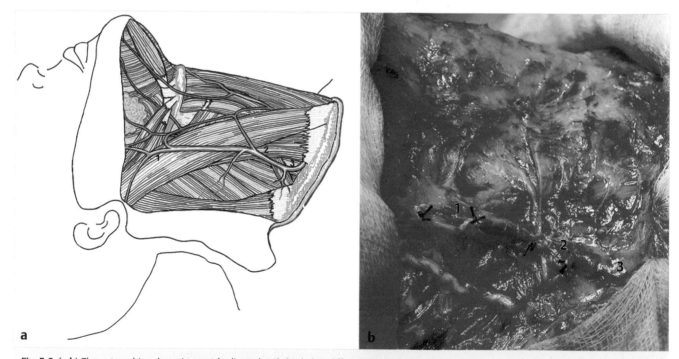

Fig. 5.6 (a,b) The external jugular vein must be ligated and divided at different levels during the operation. 1, tail of the parotid gland; 2, posterior border of the sternocleidomastoid muscle; 3, supraclavicular fossa.

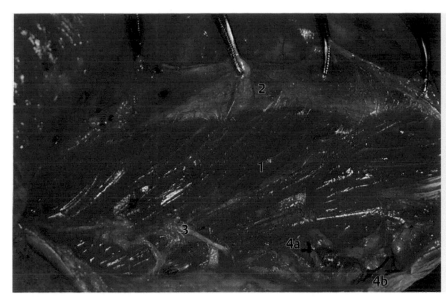

Fig. 5.7 Lateral view of the dissection of the sternocleidomastoid muscle on the right side of the neck. The fascia is incised over the posterior border of the muscle (anteriorly to the great auricular nerve) and dissected forward. Note the external jugular vein ligated at the posterior border of the sternocleidomastoid muscle and above the clavicle. 1, sternocleidomastoid muscle; 2, fascia dissected from the sternocleidomastoid muscle; 3, great auricular nerve; 4, external jugular vein (4a, ligature at the posterior border of the sternocleidomastoid muscle; 4b, ligature in the supraclavicular fossa above the clavicle).

directed to distal venous stumps. Open distal venous stumps do not always actively bleed and may be responsible for air embolism.

5.6 Incision of the Fascia over the Sternocleidomastoid Muscle

To facilitate the complete dissection of the fascia surrounding the sternocleidomastoid muscle, the initial incision must be made as close to the posterior border of the muscle as possible, but preserving the great auricular nerve in the upper part of the field (▶ Fig. 5.7). The reason for this is that the fascia is more easily dissected off the sternocleidomastoid muscle in a forward direction. Making the incision close to the posterior border of the muscle leaves no remaining fascia to be dissected posteriorly and facilitates the complete isolation of the muscle from its surrounding fascia.

5.7 The Marginal Mandibular Branch of the Facial Nerve

It is cosmetically important to preserve the marginal mandibular branch of the facial nerve. The mandibular nerve courses just deep to the superficial layer of the cervical fascia but superficial to both the anterior facial vein and artery. Identification of the nerve is time consuming and may require nerve stimulation for the novice surgeon to confirm the exact location of this thin branch of the facial nerve.

It is much easier, and equally safe, to identify, ligate, and divide the anterior facial vein at the inferior border of the submandibular gland. The superior ligature, which is left long, is reflected superiorly with a hemostat; see ▶ Fig. 5.8

and Fig. 4.19. Although the mandibular nerve is usually not seen during this maneuver, it will be automatically reflected superiorly with the skin flap, thus preventing its injury.

5.8 Preserving the Submandibular Gland

As already mentioned, removal of the submandibular gland is not a routine surgical step of functional neck dissection. The gland must be included in the specimen when the location of the primary tumor dictates its removal or when metastatic disease is suspected in the submandibular triangle. In the remaining situations the submandibular gland may be preserved. This is the case with cancer of the larynx and hypopharynx, where the lymph nodes in the submandibular and submental region (area I) are usually not involved and, additionally, there is no need to approach the primary tumor through the submandibular triangle. When a submandibular gland preserving functional neck dissection is performed, the dissection of the upper border of the surgical field must be modified with respect to the procedure described in the previous chapter.

After the flaps have been raised, the submandibular gland can be seen through the superficial layer of the cervical fascia in the upper part of the surgical field. The fascia is then incised from the midline to the tail of the parotid gland, at the level of the lower border of the submandibular gland as for a gland-removing procedure, and the anterior belly of the digastric muscle is exposed; see Fig. 4.17 and Fig. 4.18. Then the facial vein is ligated and divided (▶ Fig. 5.9), reflecting upward the superior ligature to preserve the marginal mandibular branch of the facial nerve as already mentioned; see Fig. 4.19. The

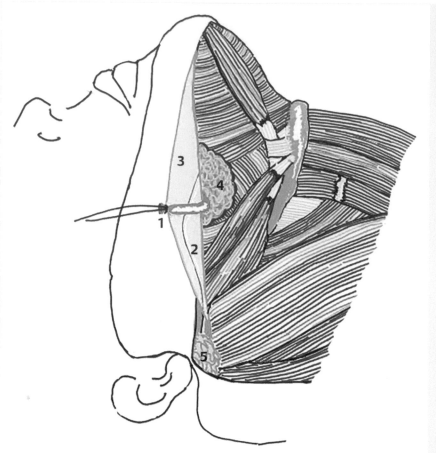

Fig. 5.8 Protection to the marginal mandibular branch of the facial nerve is obtained with the maneuver of the facial vein (right side of the neck). 1, facial vein; 2, marginal nerve; 3, fascia retracted upward; 4, submandibular gland; 5, parotid gland.

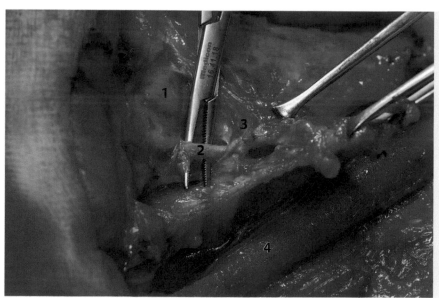

Fig. 5.9 The fascia has been incised at the inferior border of the submandibular gland and the facial vein is ligated. 1, submandibular gland; 2, facial vein; 3, fascia retracted inferiorly; 4, sternocleidomastoid muscle.

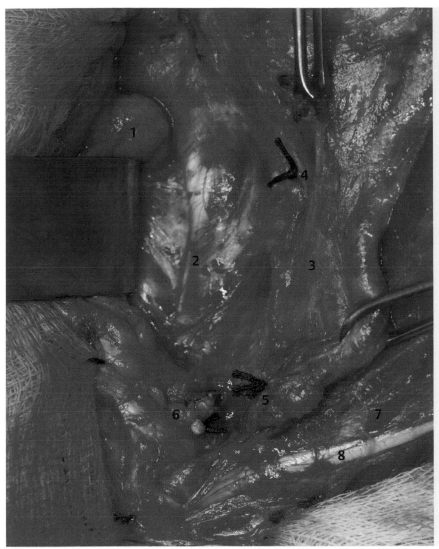

Fig. 5.10 The gland is retracted superiorly and the specimen inferiorly, exposing the digastric and stylohyoid muscles. 1, submandibular gland; 2, digastric and stylohyoid muscles; 3, specimen; 4, facial vein (proximal stump); 5, external jugular vein (ligated and divided); 6, parotid gland; 7, sternocleidomastoid muscle; 8, great auricular nerve.

retromandibular vein and the external jugular vein are also ligated and divided.

Now, instead of including the submandibular gland within the specimen, the specimen is dissected inferiorly while the gland is retracted superiorly (▶ Fig. 5.10). The dissection then continues over the digastric and stylohyoid muscles (▶ Fig. 5.11). The muscles are retracted superiorly along with the gland, and the contents of the submandibular fossa are now exposed (▶ Fig. 5.12). The fibrofatty tissue containing the upper jugular nodes is grasped and dissected off this area, preserving the gland. The dissection may be continued medially to include the submental nodes, but this is seldom required in tumors that allow preservation of the submandibular gland.

The dissection is continued inferiorly in the usual way, the only difference being the preservation of the submandibular gland.

5.9 The Lingual Veins and the Hypoglossal Nerve

The hypoglossal nerve in the submandibular triangle is crossed by a variable number of lingual veins that drain the lingual area toward the internal jugular vein (▶ Fig. 5.13). The anatomical distribution of these lingual veins is unpredictable, thus preventing a systematic approach to the area. These veins are a frequent source of troublesome bleeding because of their thin wall and the proximity to the main trunk of the hypoglossal nerve. This area must be approached carefully; it is important to avoid the placement of clamps and ligatures without clear identification of the hypoglossal nerve. Bipolar coagulation may be useful at this stage of the operation.

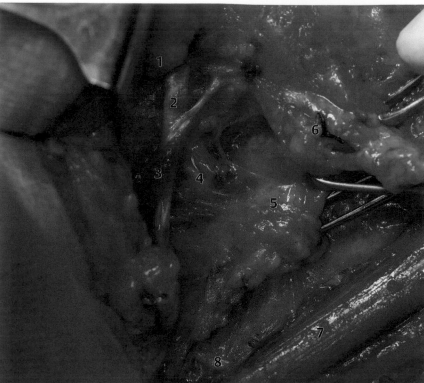

Fig. 5.11 The digastric and stylohyoid muscles have been completely dissected.
1, submandibular gland (retracted);
2, intermediate tendon of the digastric muscle;
3, stylohyoid muscle; 4, hypoglossal nerve;
5, specimen (retracted inferiorly); 6, facial vein (proximal stump); 7, sternocleidomastoid muscle;
8, spinal accessory nerve.

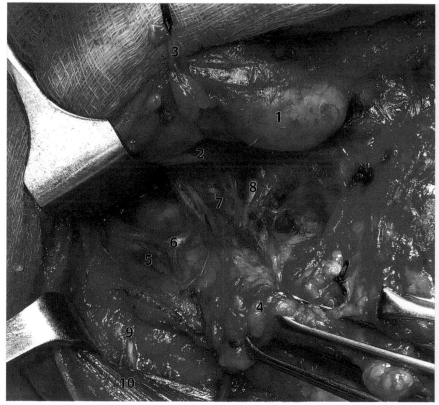

Fig. 5.12 Retraction of the submandibular gland and digastric muscle allows the dissection of the upper jugular chain. 1, submandibular gland;
2, digastric and stylohyoid muscles (retracted);
3, facial vein (distal stump); 4, specimen;
5, internal jugular vein; 6, occipital artery;
7, external carotid artery; 8, hypoglossal nerve;
9, spinal accessory nerve;
10, sternocleidomastoid muscle.

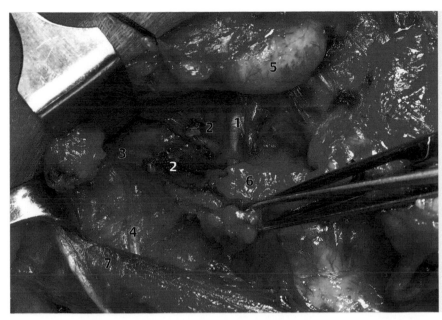

Fig. 5.13 The lingual veins have been ligated or coagulated, exposing the hypoglossal nerve completely. 1, hypoglossal nerve; 2, lingual veins; 3, internal jugular vein; 4, spinal accessory nerve; 5, submandibular gland; 6, specimen; 7, sternocleidomastoid muscle.

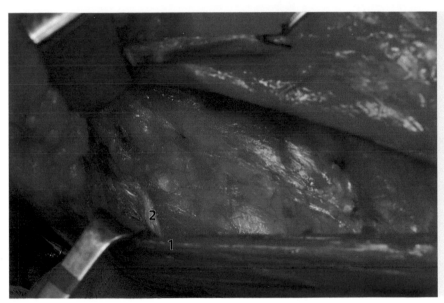

Fig. 5.14 The spinal accessory nerve is identified as it enters the sternocleidomastoid muscle. 1, sternocleidomastoid muscle; 2, spinal accessory nerve.

5.10 Identification of the Spinal Accessory Nerve

The most common complaint after radical neck dissection is the discomfort of shoulder droop resulting from spinal accessory nerve transection. Functional neck dissection preserves the spinal accessory nerve. However, shoulder function after functional neck dissection is not always normal. The explanation to this apparently paradoxical fact must be sought in the variable innervation of the shoulder, especially with respect to the participation of the cervical plexus in shoulder motility. Injury to the motor branches of the cervical plexus that supply the deep muscles of the neck may explain the variation in the degree of disability of the shoulder after preservation of the spinal accessory nerve. The possibility of motor supply to the trapezius from the cervical plexus in human beings is still controversial and rests upon indirect embryological, surgical, and clinical evidence.

The spinal accessory nerve must be identified as it enters the sternocleidomastoid muscle; see ▶ Fig. 5.14 and Fig. 4.16. This point is usually located at the junction of the upper one-third and lower two-thirds of the muscle. During the dissection of the medial aspect of the fascia of the sternocleidomastoid muscle, the entrance of the spinal accessory nerve into the muscle is easily identified. The nerve is usually accompanied by a satellite vessel that must be carefully cauterized to avoid excessive nerve stimulation.

Once identified at its entrance in the sternocleidomastoid muscle, the nerve is followed superiorly toward the internal jugular vein; see Fig. 4.27 and Fig. 4.28. The spinal accessory nerve usually comes obliquely in a posterior and inferior direction from the jugular foramen. The relations between the spinal accessory nerve and the internal jugular vein are variable. In approximately two-thirds of cases, the nerve crosses superficial to the vein. In the remaining cases, the nerve passes behind the vein (▶ Fig. 5.15) or even across it (▶ Fig. 5.16). The surgeon must keep this important information in mind while dissecting the spinal accessory nerve toward the internal jugular vein. When the vein is approached, precise identification of its wall is mandatory before complete isolation of the nerve is accomplished. Otherwise, the internal jugular vein may be easily injured.

The isolation of the spinal accessory nerve in this region takes place through the fibrofatty tissue of the upper jugular area where the scalpel is not very effective. Thus, the scissors are recommended for this step of the operation. For a satisfactory removal of all fibrofatty tissue in this area, it is important to completely isolate the spinal accessory nerve from the surrounding tissue. This will facilitate the delivery of the tissue beneath the nerve by means of the spinal accessory maneuver.

On a comprehensive functional approach, the spinal accessory nerve may also be found in the posterior triangle of the neck. At this level, the surgical position of

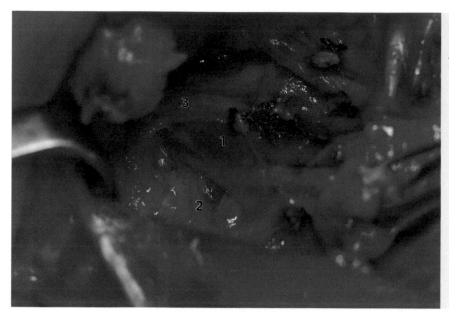

Fig. 5.15 Lateral view of the right spinal accessory nerve crossing posterior to the internal jugular vein. 1, internal jugular vein; 2, spinal accessory nerve; 3, occipital artery.

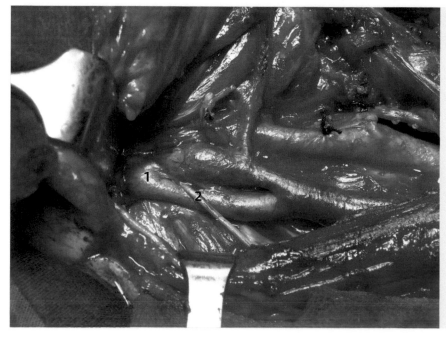

Fig. 5.16 Lateral view of the right spinal accessory nerve piercing the internal jugular vein. 1, internal jugular vein; 2, spinal accessory nerve.

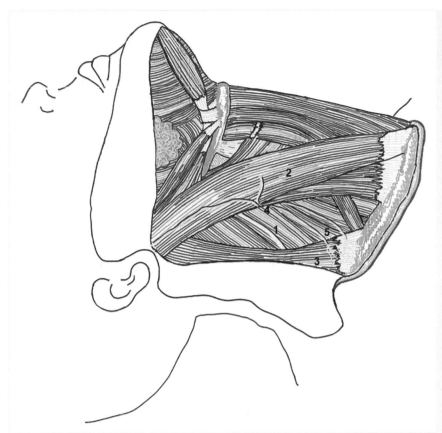

Fig. 5.17 Relations between the spinal accessory nerve and the branches of the cervical plexus within the posterior triangle of the neck. 1, spinal accessory nerve; 2, sternocleidomastoid muscle; 3, trapezius muscle; 4, Erb's point; 5, supraclavicular branches of the cervical plexus.

the patient and the traction applied to the dissected tissue may displace the nerve from its original course. Usually, a slight anterior curvature is created through the neural anastomosis of the spinal accessory nerve with the second, third, and fourth cervical nerves. To avoid injuring the spinal accessory nerve in the posterior triangle, a thorough knowledge of its anatomy is essential.

The spinal accessory nerve enters the supraclavicular triangle at its upper angle, deep to Erb's point, and descends obliquely in a posterior and inferior direction toward the trapezius muscle; see Fig. 2.22. Its course is usually associated with the posterior border of the levator scapulae muscle. The spinal accessory nerve should not be confused with several supraclavicular branches of the cervical plexus that follow a similar but more superficial course; see ▶ Fig. 5.17 and Fig. 4.37. Although it is usually not necessary, the novice surgeon may find electric stimulation useful to confirm the location of the spinal accessory nerve in the posterior triangle.

5.11 The Spinal Accessory Maneuver

Osvaldo Suárez used the term *spinal accessory maneuver* to refer to the surgical step in which the fibrofatty tissue surrounding the spinal accessory nerve in the upper jugular region is passed beneath the nerve to be removed

in-continuity with the rest of the specimen; see ▶ Fig. 5.18 and Fig. 4.31.

After the spinal accessory nerve has been completely isolated on its course from the sternocleidomastoid muscle to the internal jugular vein, the tissue lying posterior and superior to the nerve is dissected from the splenius capitis and levator scapulae muscles (▶ Fig. 5.18a). Once dissected from the plane of the deep muscles, the tissue is passed underneath the nerve to be removed en bloc with the rest of the specimen (▶ Fig. 5.18b). At this moment, two more hints may help the forthcoming dissection:

1. The tissue that has been passed beneath the nerve should also be freed from the uppermost part of the internal jugular vein (▶ Fig. 5.18b, ▶ Fig. 5.19). This facilitates the dissection of the carotid sheath on a later step of the operation.

2. After the spinal accessory maneuver has been completed, the dissection is continued anterior to the sternocleidomastoid muscle in a downward direction for a few more centimeters. Keeping the sternocleidomastoid muscle retracted posteriorly, a number-10 knife blade is used to cut the tissue located below the entrance of spinal accessory nerve, until the underlying levator scapulae muscle is noted (▶ Fig. 5.19, ▶ Fig. 5.20). This cut is taken inferiorly to the level of Erb's point, and helps in the dissection of the deep muscles that will be performed on a later step of the operation.

5

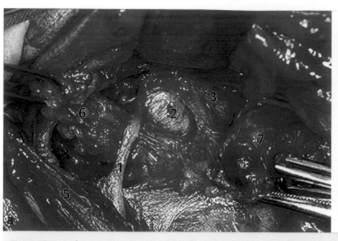 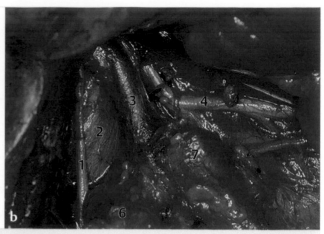

Fig. 5.18 Spinal accessory maneuver on the right side of the neck. (**a**) The fibrofatty tissue of the upper spinal accessory region has been dissected from the deep muscular floor. (**b**) The dissected tissue has been passed beneath the nerve to join the specimen coming from the submandibular area. 1, spinal accessory nerve; 2, levator scapulae muscle; 3, internal jugular vein; 4, hypoglossal nerve; 5, sternocleidomastoid muscle; 6, specimen from the upper spinal accessory region; 7, specimen from the upper jugular and submandibular area.

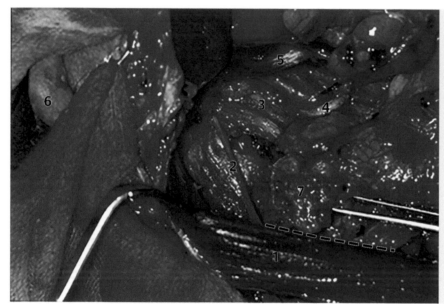

Fig. 5.19 The spinal accessory maneuver is completed and the specimen has been dissected from the upper part of the internal jugular vein on the right side of the neck. A final cut is made below the spinal accessory nerve (*dashed line*). 1, sternocleidomastoid muscle; 2, spinal accessory nerve; 3, internal jugular vein; 4, hypoglossal nerve; 5, digastric muscle; 6, ear lobule; 7, specimen from the upper jugular and spinal accessory area.

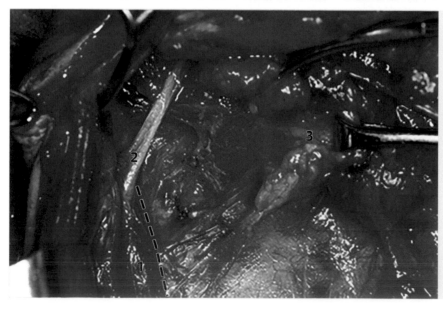

Fig. 5.20 Before approaching the supraclavicular area, a final downward cut is made anterior to the sternocleidomastoid muscle (*dashed line*). This cut extends approximately 2 cm below the spinal accessory nerve and should be carried deep to the levator scapulae muscle. 1, sternocleidomastoid muscle; 2, spinal accessory nerve; 3, specimen from the upper spinal accessory region.

5.12 The Transverse Cervical Vessels

The transverse cervical artery and vein constitute important anatomical landmarks in the posterior triangle of the neck. The transverse cervical artery is one of the branches of the thyrocervical trunk. The variations in the branches and the exact manner of branching of the thyrocervical trunk are numerous; see Fig. 4.39. However, the prevailing patterns usually show at least one branch that runs almost transversely across the neck, anterior to the anterior scalene muscle and the brachial plexus (▶ Fig. 5.21).

The transverse cervical artery is usually accompanied by a vein. Both are found within the fibrofatty tissue of the supraclavicular fossa and often may be preserved during functional neck dissection. However, there is an inconstant ascending branch from the thyrocervical trunk that usually must be ligated and divided to allow a complete dissection of the supraclavicular fossa. This ascending cervical artery may arise from the inferior thyroid artery or from other arteries at the base of the neck, and it is frequently represented by more than one vessel.

5.13 Preserving the Branches of the Cervical Plexus

As already mentioned, the cervical plexus has important connections to the spinal accessory nerve. A branch from the second cervical nerve typically joins the spinal accessory nerve before it enters the sternocleidomastoid muscle. Also, branches from the second, third, and fourth cervical nerves join the spinal accessory nerve (▶ Fig. 5.22). Although the branches connecting the cervical plexus with the spinal accessory nerve are believed to

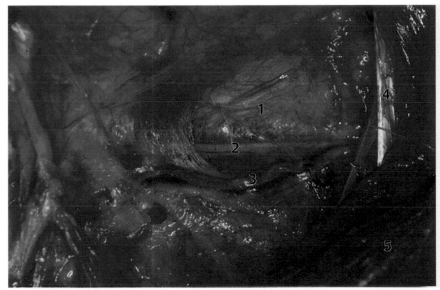

Fig. 5.21 Right supraclavicular fossa after removal of its lymphatic contents. 1, carotid sheath; 2, phrenic nerve; 3, transverse cervical vessels; 4, omohyoid muscle; 5, sternocleidomastoid muscle.

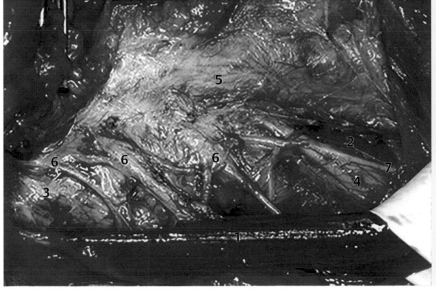

Fig. 5.22 The deep branches of the cervical plexus have been preserved on the right side of the neck. 1, sternocleidomastoid muscle; 2, anterior scalene muscle; 3, levator scapulae muscle; 4, brachial plexus; 5, carotid sheath; 6, deep branches of the cervical plexus; 7, phrenic nerve.

be sensory, surgical evidence suggests that their preservation results in better shoulder function.

A thorough knowledge of the anatomy of the cervical plexus is necessary to preserve the connecting branches with the spinal accessory nerve. The cervical plexus is formed by the ventral rami of the second, third, and fourth cervical nerves, and also sometimes with a contribution from the first (see Chapter 2). This neural network has two types of branches, superficial or cutaneous, and deep. The superficial branches arise from a series of loops between the second, third, and fourth cervical nerves. The most constant are the lesser occipital, the great auricular, the transverse cervical, and the supraclavicular nerves. Some of these sensory branches will be transected during the operation.

On the other hand, the deep branches are largely motor, except for the contribution to the sternocleidomastoid and trapezius muscles, where controversy still remains. The deep branches include the ansa hypoglossi, or ansa cervicalis (▶ Fig. 5.23), the phrenic nerve (▶ Fig. 5.21), and the branches to the deep cervical muscles (▶ Fig. 5.22). Except for the ansa cervicalis, whose traject is different, the deep branches of the cervical plexus should be preserved by keeping the dissection superficial to their course. The anterior cervical nerves should be sectioned distal to the point where the deep branches leave the main root; see Fig. 4.42. The motor supply to the levator scapulae muscle can also be preserved by staying superficial to the deep layer of the cervical fascia at the level of the midportion of the levator scapulae. This is where the neurovascular supply enters the muscle.

5.14 Preserving the Phrenic Nerve

The phrenic nerve is a deep branch of the cervical plexus with neural contribution from the brachial plexus. It usually arises from the third, fourth, and fifth cervical nerves; see Fig. 2.25. The nerve courses downward with a slight medial inclination over the anterior face of the anterior scalene muscle. It runs directly on the anterior surface of the muscle fibers, between them and the overlying fascia, which is the prevertebral layer of the cervical fascia (▶ Fig. 5.21, ▶ Fig. 5.22); see also Fig. 4.40. The phrenic nerve provides motor function to the ipsilateral diaphragm.

The easiest way to avoid injuring the phrenic nerve is to stay superficial to the prevertebral layer of the cervical fascia at the level of the anterior scalene muscle. This will keep the phrenic nerve protected by the fascial layer. When approaching the carotid sheath, the anterior superficial branches of the cervical plexus must be transected distal to the exit of the phrenic roots to preserve the deep cervical contributions and maintain the anatomical and functional integrity of the phrenic nerve.

5.15 The Sympathetic Trunk

The cervical sympathetic chain consists of several ganglia, between two and four, and the trunk connecting them. The sympathetic trunk lies medial to the phrenic nerve and posterior to the carotid sheath. It may be found during the dissection of the carotid sheath, when the surgeon carries the dissection too far medially over the deep muscles; see ▶ Fig. 5.24 and Fig. 4.44. In these cases, it may be mistaken for the vagus nerve when, in reality, the vagus nerve runs more anteriorly within the carotid sheath, not posterior to it, between the carotid artery and the internal jugular vein. Precise knowledge of the anatomy of this area is important to prevent injury to the sympathetic trunk.

The basic references for identifying the sympathetic trunk are its close relation to the posterior wall of the carotid artery and its medial situation with respect to other neural neck structures. Unlike the phrenic nerve, the

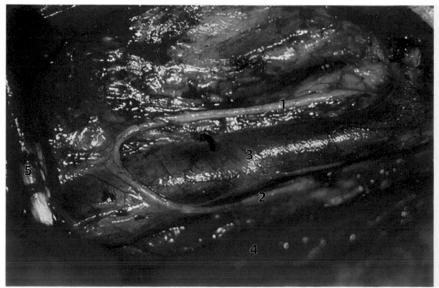

Fig. 5.23 Ansa cervicalis on the left side of the neck. 1, superior root of the ansa cervicalis; 2, inferior root of the ansa cervicalis; 3, internal jugular vein; 4, sternocleidomastoid muscle; 5, omohyoid muscle.

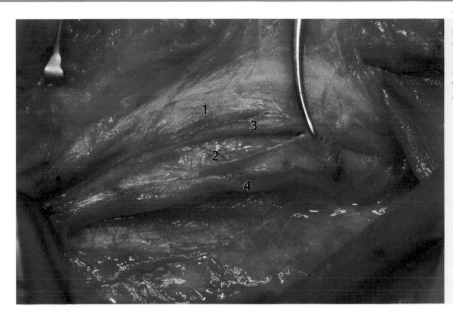

Fig. 5.24 The sympathetic trunk lies posterior to the carotid sheath, whereas the vagus nerve runs between the internal jugular vein and the carotid artery (right side of the neck). 1, internal jugular vein; 2, carotid artery; 3, vagus nerve; 4, sympathetic trunk (retracted with the fascia).

5

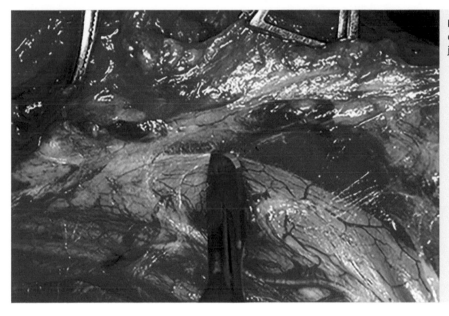

Fig. 5.25 Adequate positioning of the scalpel is crucial for a safe dissection over the internal jugular vein.

sympathetic trunk does not lie upon the anterior scalene muscle, but medial to it.

5.16 Danger Points in the Dissection of the Internal Jugular Vein

Preservation of the internal jugular vein is one of the main advantages of functional neck dissection. Under normal conditions this is not a difficult step of the operation. However, some particular details may contribute to a successful dissection of this important structure.

We prefer the scalpel for this part of the operation, which is usually striking given its apparent "danger." However, it is our experience that, if properly performed,

knife dissection of the carotid sheath is the most effective, clean, and safe way to dissect the lymphatic tissue in this area.

The general rules for safe knife dissection that have been previously described in this chapter must be carefully followed. Adequate tension must be applied to all tissues. Gentle movements must be performed by the surgeon and surrounding personnel. The knife blade must be directed obliquely against the wall of the internal jugular vein (▶ Fig. 5.25). And, finally, the entire length of the vein must be dissected in a continuous fashion, from the clavicle to the mastoid.

In spite of all these measures, two danger points are usually found at the beginning of every dissection of the carotid sheath. They correspond to both ends of the dissected internal jugular vein. We refer to these points as the "two initial folds" because here the vein wall folds as a consequence of the traction exerted by the dissected tissue (▶ Fig. 5.26, ▶ Fig. 5.27). Before further dissection of the carotid sheath is accomplished, these two folds should be carefully removed without injuring the internal jugular vein. It is important to know that the folded wall of the vein is especially sensible to the cutting edge of sharp instruments (scissors, scalpel). Thus, extreme care must be taken when working in these areas.

The upper fold may be less marked if the tissue from the upper spinal accessory nerve region was previously dissected off the wall of the internal jugular vein as described during the spinal accessory maneuver (▶ Fig. 5.18b, ▶ Fig. 5.19, ▶ Fig. 5.26). The lower fold is usually located at the level of the crossing between the omohyoid muscle and the internal jugular vein (▶ Fig. 5.27a). In fact, the omohyoid muscle greatly contributes to this fold. Thus, if the omohyoid muscle is to be removed with the primary tumor, it can be transected at this moment to help the

dissection of the lower part of the carotid sheath. On the other hand, when the omohyoid muscle is to be preserved, inferior retraction of the muscle allows better exposure of the lower part of the internal jugular vein and facilitates the dissection of the lower fold (▶ Fig. 5.27b).

After both ends of the internal jugular vein have been freed, the dissection must be carried along the entire length of the vein, cutting obliquely with the scalpel over the tense wall of the vein. As the medial aspect of the vein is approached, several tributaries may be identified. The smaller veins can be cauterized, taking care not to injure the wall of the internal jugular vein, whereas the larger trunks need to be ligated and divided (▶ Fig. 5.28).

5.17 The Thoracic Duct

The large lymphatic channels that terminate at the base of the neck are the thoracic duct on the left side and the right

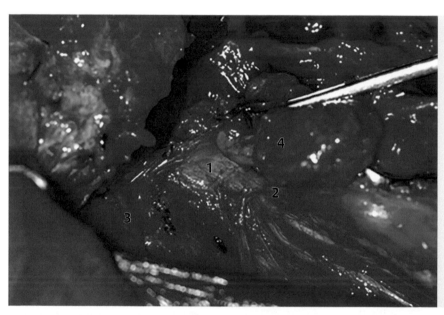

Fig. 5.26 Upper fold of the carotid sheath at the internal jugular vein on the right side of the neck. To facilitate the dissection at this level, the tissue was dissected off the upper part of the internal jugular vein at the end of the spinal accessory maneuver. 1, internal jugular vein; 2, upper fold; 3, spinal accessory nerve; 4, specimen from the upper spinal accessory region.

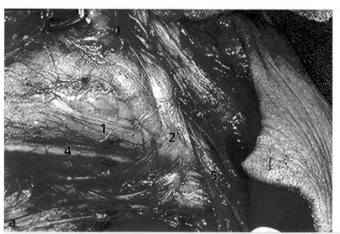

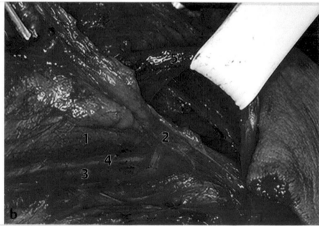

Fig. 5.27 Danger points in the dissection of the carotid sheath. Lower fold over the internal jugular vein on the right side of the neck. (a) The lower fold develops at the crossing of the omohyoid muscle and the internal jugular vein. (b) Retraction of the omohyoid muscle facilitates the dissection of the lower fold. 1, internal jugular vein; 2, lower fold; 3, carotid artery; 4, vagus nerve; 5, omohyoid muscle.

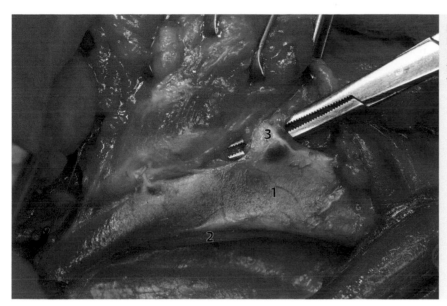

Fig. 5.28 Middle thyroid vein draining into the internal jugular vein on the right side of the neck. 1, internal jugular vein; 2, vagus nerve; 3, middle thyroid vein draining into the internal jugular vein.

lymphatic duct on the right side (see Fig. 4.50). The right lymphatic duct is not a common source of problems during neck dissection. However, injuring the thoracic duct during the operation results in persistent chylous leak that may be extremely difficult to solve in patients with a functional approach. Preservation of the sternocleidomastoid muscle in these patients decreases the efficacy of the usual compressive maneuvers that are used to stop chylous leak. Thus, early recognition of lymphatic leakage during the operation is crucial in order to repair the injury before closure. Precise knowledge of the cervical course of the thoracic duct is fundamental to avoid postoperative problems.

The exact end point of the thoracic duct is variable because it may open into the internal jugular vein, the subclavian vein, or the angle of junction between them. Also, the termination of the duct may be doubled, tripled, or even quadrupled. All these variations, along with the frail thin walls of the duct, facilitate its injury at surgery.

The best way to avoid injuring the thoracic duct is by not approaching the base of the neck on the left side unless it is absolutely necessary. When the operation must proceed to the lowest part of the left side of the neck, the surgeon must be aware of the variable anatomy of the thoracic duct when approaching the junction of the internal jugular and subclavian veins. If the duct is to be ligated to include in the dissection the tissue at the level of the final portion of the internal jugular vein, additional tissue must be included in the ligature to avoid sectioning the thin wall of the thoracic duct with the suture. Thus, the area of the duct is surrounded by muscle, fascia, or adipose tissue before being sutured with 3–0 atraumatic silk.

When the duct is inadvertently sectioned, the lymph drains overtly at the base of the neck. This situation must be recognized and repaired during the operation. The typical transparent, slightly yellow liquid with particles of fat positively identifies the presence of lymphorrhea from a sectioned thoracic duct. In such instances the ruptured opening of the duct must be identified and repaired, including additional tissue in the ligature, as mentioned before. It is not uncommon after involuntary section of the thoracic duct that the open end of the vessel cannot be identified. In these cases, the area where the lymph appears at the base of the neck must be sutured, including enough tissue to stop the leak. Attentive examination of the area must be performed after repair to assure the cessation of the leak. Asking the anesthetist to momentarily increase the thoracic pressure may help in the identification of the cut end of the duct and to assess the resolution of the lymphorrhea.

Although the right lymphatic duct is seldom a problem, the same principles must be applied in case of a right chylous leak.

6 Complications of Neck Surgery

6.1 Introduction

Postoperative complications after neck surgery have a significant impact on morbidity and health care cost, leading to prolonged hospitalizations, further operations, permanent sequelae, and sometimes, fatal outcome. Aging, poor nutritional status, and chronic diseases of the respiratory, cardiovascular, and other systems (due to alcohol and tobacco abuse) are common factors in most patients with tumors of the upper aerodigestive tract. Salvage surgery after chemo-radiation protocols is currently a major source of severe complications.

Concerning neck dissection, it is difficult to identify the complications directly related to the procedure and separate them from those associated with removal of the primary tumor because both surgeries are usually performed at the same time. The complications that can be more specifically related to neck dissection and will be addressed in this chapter are as follows.

Cervical complications associated with functional and selective neck dissection include the following:

- Local complications:
  - Infection.
  - Serohematoma.
  - Wound dehiscence.
  - Chylous fistula.
- Vascular complications:
  - Hemorrhage.
  - Vascular blowout.
- Neural complications:
  - Spinal accessory nerve.
  - Phrenic nerve.
  - Hypoglossal nerve.
  - Vagus nerve.
  - Recurrent laryngeal nerve.
  - Sympathetic trunk.
  - Mandibular branch of cranial nerve VII.
  - Brachial plexus.

General complications associated with functional and selective neck dissection include:

- Pulmonary complications:
  - Pneumonia.
  - Pulmonary embolism.
- Stress ulcer.
- Sepsis.
- Hypoparathyroidism.
- Other.

6.2 Cervical Complications

6.2.1 Local Complications

Infection and Serohematoma

Infection following functional and selective neck dissection is unusual, around 3%, and frequently related to hematoma. Infection is more frequent when the neck dissection is associated with surgical procedures that include opening of the aerodigestive tract. The majority of wound infections are related to pharyngocutaneous fistula after laryngectomy. Infection is best prevented by meticulous sterile surgical technique, gentle handling of the tissue, irrigation, and adequate placing of suction catheters. Necrotic tissue, in the form of residue after either ligature or coagulation, is a focus for bacterial growth. Suction catheter minimizes the incidence of hematoma and seroma, which are frequently associated with wound infection by constituting an ideal media for bacterial growth.

Hematoma and seroma are usually due to inadequate hemostasis at the time of surgery, coagulation disorders, drain obstruction, or incorrect placement of drains. Any effective measure that prevents dead space and hematoma is also useful in minimizing infection. We usually place one suction catheter on each side of the neck after neck dissection. Correct functioning of the drain should be checked immediately after surgery and periodically during the early postoperative period. Inadequate suture of the trachea to the skin in patients requiring tracheostomy results in a cervical opening that prevents vacuum, leading to blood collection and eventually infection, when suction drains are used. The drain is removed on the second or third postoperative day, depending on the output. If seroma develops in spite of these maneuvers, it can be evacuated by needle aspiration, drained through the wound, or observed for gradual absorption. However, prompt drainage will decrease the chances of bacterial contamination.

In procedures not requiring opening of the aerodigestive tract, functional neck dissection is considered a clean surgical procedure, and perioperative antibiotics are not beneficial in preventing infection. Antibiotic prophylaxis is important to decrease the infection rate in some surgical procedures, although it is not the key to the problem in isolated neck dissection. Different antibiotic combinations that cover aerobic and anaerobic bacteria are reported depending on the individual preferences. Dose, time of administration, and type of antibiotic depend on personal preferences and are different at each institution.

Infection should be suspected in a patient with spiking fever, chills, malaise, odor, and swelling or edema of the skin flaps. A small separate incision, or the opening of a limited window in the skin incision, is usually sufficient to drain a serohematoma and prevent further elevation of the flaps with the risk of necrosis and exposure of the great vessels.

Wound Dehiscence

Wound dehiscence is related to inadequate planning of the incision or to infection. Proper placement of the incision should be planned before surgery. The location of the incision and its length should be sufficient to allow adequate exposure to minimize the need for vigorous wound retraction intraoperatively. The skin flaps should be carefully protected from retractors or cautery. We usually fix wet towels to the skin flaps to protect the skin throughout the operation and to avoid direct traction over the skin edge. Crosshatch marks should be avoided to improve the cosmetic results and to avoid additional scarring. Methylene blue or surgical pen marks allow proper realignment of long incisions during skin closure without the risk of additional scars.

In previously irradiated patients, careful skin realignment and subcutaneous suture are important to avoid wound dehiscence facilitated by radiation-induced devascularization. When the patient has been heavily irradiated and the skin is atrophic, it is better to use mattress sutures, placing a rubber catheter between the suture and the skin to decrease tension with subsequent ischemia and skin necrosis.

Chylous Fistula

Chylous leakage is an uncommon complication, with a reported incidence of 1 to 2.5%. It is much more frequent on the left side of the neck. When the thoracic duct is to be ligated during surgery, it should be surrounded by muscle, fascia, or adipose tissue to avoid sectioning its thin wall with the ligature. After ligation, the lower part of the left side of the neck must be carefully inspected for chyle pooling. Asking the anesthesiologist to increase the intrathoracic pressure and placing the patient in the Trendelenburg position are helpful in the intraoperative identification of chyle leak in the area of the thoracic duct. It is important to note that in most patients developing postoperative chyle fistula, this was previously identified and apparently controlled intraoperatively.

In the postoperative period, chylous fistula is recognized by the appearance of a milky fluid in the drains. This is usually evident within the first 5 days after surgery. The chylous origin of the fluid can be confirmed by measuring the content of triglycerides, usually over 100 mg/dL. When chylous leak is suspected, dietary modifications can be prescribed. Low fat diet, either enteral or parenteral, is usually recommended because medium-chain triglycerides are absorbed directly into the portal venous circulation, avoiding the thoracic duct. Elevation of the head, repeated aspiration, and pressure dressing are also recommended. It is important to note, however, that preservation of the sternocleidomastoid muscle in functional and selective neck dissection constitutes an important obstacle for successful compression. The daily volume of the leak has been reported to range from 80 to 4,500 mL. When more than 500 mL of chyle drain per day, nonsurgical stop is unlikely.

If no response is found upon conservative treatment, the lower part of the neck should be surgically explored. Before surgery is attempted it may be helpful to put the patient on a high lipid enteral diet to give chyle a thick and milky consistency, which will improve the intraoperative identification of the leak.

6.2.2 Vascular Complications

Bleeding

Bleeding is not a frequent complication after neck dissection, but when it happens, it is important to determine whether the hemorrhage is due to a small superficial vessel or to a more important deep vessel. Superficial bleeding is usually bright red, it does not bulge the skin flaps, and it tends to stop with gentle external compression or by placing a stitch around the bleeding point. Generalized oozing of blood can produce up to 500 mL in a few hours. On the other hand, ballooning of the skin flaps or filling the drain system containers with more than 250 mL of blood in less than 30 minutes indicates a more serious hemorrhage.

In our experience, the most frequent sources of venous bleeding after functional and selective neck dissection are the retromandibular vein at the tail of the parotid gland, the branches of the transverse cervical vein in the supraclavicular fossa, and small veins draining into the internal jugular vein. When the tail of the parotid gland is included in the resection, the retromandibular vein should be identified and ligated. Dissection of area IV and the lower part of area V may result in inadvertent sectioning of small branches of the transverse cervical vein. When the patient's blood pressure is low, the inferior stump of the transected vein may retract caudally without bleeding during the operation. Then, when the patient wakes up from the anesthesia, cough and increased abdominal pressure may induce bleeding. The same may happen when small branches of the internal jugular vein are sectioned during the dissection of the carotid sheath, especially those located on the posterior aspect of the vein.

To identify any possible source of venous bleeding not detected during the operation, it is important to wash the surgical field with saline at the end of the operation and ask the anesthetist to increase the venous pressure to force bleeding from unnoticed opened veins. When hemoclips are used during the operation, care must be taken while cleaning to avoid unintentional displacement of the clips, leaving a collapsed vessel that can eventually bleed with a sudden increase in venous pressure. On the other hand, the small veins draining directly into the internal jugular vein are better ligated than cauterized, especially when they are to be sectioned close to the wall of the internal jugular vein because necrosis induced by the cautery may produce hemorrhage in the late postoperative period. Special attention should be paid to electrocautery in previously irradiated patients.

Arterial bleeding is more evident at surgery than venous bleeding. It is usually secondary to malposition or displacement of a ligature. The most frequent sources of arterial bleeding in our experience are the superior laryngeal pedicle and the inferior thyroid artery.

When hemorrhage is suspected in the immediate postoperative period, adequate blood replacement and airway maintenance should be ensured as first priority. Then, the patient should be taken to the operating room where the neck should be explored under aseptic conditions with good illumination and adequate material. Evacuation of blood clots and hematoma, along with washing the surgical field, helps in identifying the bleeding vessels and reduces the risk of infection. The use of compressive dressing is not recommended because, although it may reduce postoperative edema, it does not stop the development of hematoma, and may in fact delay its recognition.

6.2.3 Vascular Blowout

In most cases, this dramatic complication is not related to neck dissection but to other problems associated with surgery for the primary tumor, especially pharyngocutaneous fistula. This complication is typical in patients surgically treated for laryngeal and hypopharyngeal carcinomas. Continuous leakage of saliva into the wound may produce secondary infection and necrosis, which eventually may lead to a blowout of any of the major vessels in the neck. Other factors such as malnutrition, diabetes, and previous radiation therapy increase the risk of vascular blowout by increasing the risk of local infection and fistula formation. Any bleeding from the wound should be considered an alert sign. If bleeding persists and a pharyngocutaneous fistula is present, then surgical exploration of the neck is recommended.

Vascular blowout is especially serious when it affects the carotid artery. This is an often-fatal complication and a terrible experience for the patient, the family, and the treatment team. On the other hand, the internal jugular vein blowout, although serious, seldom has a fatal outcome. Rupture of the internal jugular vein is often preceded by previous hemorrhage of lower intensity. No attempt should be made to control the hemorrhage at bedside by placing hemostats because this maneuver usually produces further rupture of the vessel, mainly in those cases associated with infection secondary to pharyngocutaneous fistula. The airway must be ensured, a good intravenous fluid line should be used, and blood samples for cross-matching should be obtained while pressure is maintained over the vessel. Control of massive bleeding from the carotid artery or the internal jugular vein should be attempted in the operating room with adequate personnel, monitoring, and surgical material.

The carotid artery should be explored caudal first, until a normal artery is found. The risk of neurological sequelae from ligation of the common carotid artery must be accepted because its repair is seldom possible due to the lack of normal walls in the proximity of the ruptured area. On the other hand, ligation of the internal jugular vein on one side has no important side effects, even after bilateral procedures, because the patency of the contralateral vein ensures acceptable blood drainage. The situation changes when both veins are ligated simultaneously. Facial and cerebral edema can dramatically appear within a few hours after surgery and must be combated by positioning the patient at 45 degrees, avoiding pressure dressing, checking fluid and electrolyte balance, and monitoring central venous pressure. Cerebral edema is a serious complication, producing progressive neurological deficit that may lead to coma. It requires careful management by taking the patient to the intensive care unit until normal circulation is regained. Long-lasting facial edema may be alleviated by frequent massage that contributes to the development of collateral circulation. This maneuver is especially important in previously irradiated patients in whom normal circulation is further impaired as a result of radiotherapy.

6.2.4 Neural Complications

Spinal Accessory Nerve

Dysfunction of the spinal accessory nerve and subsequent shoulder pain after radical neck dissection is one of the reasons that led to less aggressive techniques for the management of neck metastasis in head-and-neck cancer patients. Unfortunately, preservation of the nerve does not always mean nerve function preservation. Every effort should be made to avoid unnecessary trauma to the nerve, especially stretching or using electrocautery in its vicinity. Damage of the spinal accessory nerve produces denervation of the trapezius muscle, one of the main shoulder abductor muscles. This results in the so-called shoulder syndrome characterized by pain, weakness, deformity of the shoulder girdle, and inability to abduct the shoulder above 90 degrees.

The shoulder syndrome can appear not only after trauma to the nerve, but also when its anastomoses with the cervical plexus are severed. The role of the neural connections between the spinal accessory nerve and some deep branches of the cervical plexus has been widely debated in the literature. Although most anatomy textbooks insist on the sensory nature of these connections, surgical evidence suggests a motor participation of the cervical plexus on shoulder function. The branch of Maubrac, though not always present, may contribute to the motor supply of the shoulder. This nerve is sometimes present as a dominant branch with two or three additional smaller branches that join the spinal accessory nerve. When these nerves are visible, every effort should be made to preserve them as long as it is oncologically safe. The spinal accessory nerve frequently divides before entering the muscle, and all branches must be preserved to obtain the best shoulder function.

A study specifically focused on quality-of-life issues and pain after neck dissection with preservation or transection of the spinal accessory nerve found that patients in whom the nerve was preserved had less pain and less need for medication. Thus, although preservation of the nerve at surgery does not guarantee normal function, fewer sequelae and better results are obtained in nerve-sparing procedures.

Surgical preservation of the spinal accessory nerve is best accomplished if the nerve is located before further manipulation is carried out in the area. This is a general policy that should be carefully followed in every surgical procedure. As in warfare, the key to surgical success is "finding the enemy before the enemy finds us." The first place to look for the nerve is at its entrance into the sternocleidomastoid muscle. This usually happens on the medial surface of the upper third of the sternocleidomastoid muscle, close to its posterior border. A number of small vessels usually accompany the nerve at this point. It is important to avoid blind placement of hemostats and careless monopolar cautery in the vicinity of the nerve. Bipolar coagulation may be used in this area to decrease the risk of nerve damage.

Sometimes the anatomical features of the neck or special tumor conditions may obstruct the identification of the spinal accessory nerve at its entrance into the sternocleidomastoid muscle. On these occasions, the search must be taken medially to identify the nerve where it crosses the internal jugular vein. This usually happens with the nerve running superficial to the vein at the level of the lateral process of the atlas. However, it is not unusual to see the nerve crossing posterior to the vein or even across it (Fig. 2.21, Fig. 4.28, Fig. 5.14, Fig. 5.15, Fig. 5.16). This eventuality has been reported in 18 to 30% of cases and should be kept in mind to avoid unintentional damage to the spinal accessory nerve or to the internal jugular vein.

Identification is not the only goal of a nerve-sparing procedure. Gentle manipulation of the nerve is of the utmost importance if nerve function is to be preserved. Muscle retraction in the area of entrance of the spinal accessory nerve should be gentle to prevent nerve stretching leading to neurapraxia. It is also important not to retract the nerve along with the muscle during the dissection because this will also result in direct trauma with function impairment.

The novice surgeon is usually concerned about nerve identification at the upper part of the surgical field as previously exposed. However, this is not the most frequent place to damage the nerve during functional and selective neck dissection. The most dangerous area for injuring the spinal accessory nerve in a comprehensive neck dissection, including area V, is the vicinity of Erb's point, where the nerve leaves the sternocleidomastoid muscle toward the trapezius muscle. In this region the spinal accessory nerve is located directly underneath the skin and surrounded by fibrofatty tissue. The spinal accessory nerve leaves the sternocleidomastoid muscle approximately 1 cm deep to Erb's point and follows an imaginary line connecting the angle of the mandible with the acromion. The position of the patient's head along with the traction exerted by the surgeon during the dissection may displace the nerve from its original course, creating a slight anterior curvature where the nerve may be inadvertently damaged. This displacement is due to the nerve connections with the second, third, and fourth cervical nerves. Precise knowledge of neck anatomy is crucial to avoid injuring the spinal accessory nerve in this area.

Phrenic Nerve

Injury to the phrenic nerve results in paralysis of the ipsilateral diaphragm because this nerve is the only motor supply to the muscle that is responsible for 70% of respiratory movement. There are two maneuvers during which the phrenic nerve may be injured: (1) at the dissection of the fibrofatty tissue over the scalene fascia; and (2) while sectioning the anterior branches of the cervical plexus.

The phrenic nerve runs under the fascia covering the anterior and medial surface of the anterior scalene muscle. A useful anatomical landmark for the identification of the phrenic nerve is the transverse cervical artery and vein that always cross anterior to the nerve. A frequent mistake of the novice surgeon is to include the fascia of the anterior scalene muscle in the dissection, enclosing the phrenic nerve with the specimen. To avoid this, the phrenic nerve must be identified before further dissection is performed on the area. The surgeon must remain superficial to the scalene fascia while following the transverse cervical vessels anteriorly until the phrenic nerve comes into view. Once identified, the nerve should be followed upward before transecting the anterior branches of the cervical plexus. This helps preserve the nerve roots of the phrenic nerve coming from the third, fourth, and fifth cervical nerves.

Hypoglossal Nerve

The hypoglossal nerve can be found in the upper part of the surgical field (area II) close to the jugulodigastric node, which is one of the most frequent areas of regional meta-

6

stases in head-and-neck cancer. The nerve is usually identified during the dissection of the submandibular gland where it can be seen underneath the lingual veins. These should be handled carefully because of their fragile wall. If bleeding from the lingual veins occurs near the hypoglossal nerve, blind placement of hemostats and monopolar coagulation should be avoided to prevent injury to the nerve. Bipolar coagulation must be used in this area. It is also recommended that the hypoglossal nerve be identified prior to ligation of the facial artery in the submandibular triangle.

Recurrent Laryngeal Nerve

The recurrent laryngeal nerve is at risk during thyroidectomy or central compartment dissections. The nerve should be identified during thyroidectomy some millimeters inferiorly to Berry's ligament, passing between superior and inferior parathyroid glands, and crossing the inferior thyroid artery either superficial, deep or between the final branches of the artery. Intraoperative nerve monitoring systems may help with the identification. As stated in Chapters 2 and 4, the anatomy of the recurrent laryngeal nerve is different on each side. Secondary to these differences, the right recurrent laryngeal nerve is more commonly damaged during surgery than the left one.

Recurrent laryngeal nerve damage in the central compartment produces an ipsilateral vocal cord palsy in paramedian position. When unilateral, it manifests as dysphonia (breathy, bitonal voice) and dysphagia (cough while swallowing liquids) in a variable severity. The contralateral vocal cord tends to compensate the deficit in the following days or weeks. When this compensation is not achieved spontaneously, different voice therapy techniques as well as surgical procedures may be indicated to restore voice and swallowing quality. In bilateral nerve palsy the glottal space is severely reduced, causing dyspnea and usually requiring a tracheostomy.

Vagus Nerve

The vagus nerve is widely exposed during the dissection of the carotid sheath and should be considered an important "allied" during this step of the operation. The dissection of the carotid sheath begins with a longitudinal incision over the vagus nerve that herein lies between the carotid artery and the internal jugular vein. This maneuver should be gently performed to avoid injury to the nerve. Deep incision into the carotid sheath may damage its neurovascular contents, and the fascial plane for the dissection will be lost.

Another risk area for the vagus nerve during functional and selective neck dissection is the lower part of the neck in the vicinity of the thoracic duct. When the operation requires ligation of the thoracic duct, the vagus nerve must be identified before the duct is surrounded by tissue and ligated to prevent including the nerve within the ligature.

Sympathetic Trunk

The sympathetic trunk lies deep and medial to the carotid artery. When the dissection over the deep cervical muscles is taken too far medially behind the carotid sheath, the sympathetic trunk is at risk. To avoid damaging this important neural structure, the dissection must proceed anteriorly as soon as the carotid sheath comes into view. Then, a longitudinal incision is made over the vagus nerve, along the entire length of the carotid sheath, leaving the sympathetic trunk between the prevertebral fascia and the carotid artery.

Mandibular Branch of the Facial Nerve

The mandibular branch of the facial nerve runs on the undersurface of the platysma muscle, superficial to the facial vein. It is particularly vulnerable during the elevation of the flaps as well as at the dissection of the submandibular gland. Damage to this nerve results in altered motion of the corner of the mouth as a consequence of paralysis of the orbicularis oris muscle.

As with any other nerve, the best way to avoid its damage is by precise identification before further resection is performed. However, this task is tedious due to the small size of the nerve and may expose it to unnecessary risk. There is a surgical maneuver that uses the facial vein as a landmark to protect the nerve and retract it from the surgical field; see Fig. 4.18, Fig. 4.19, and Fig. 5.8. Shortly, the facial vein is identified at the lower part of the submandibular gland, where it is ligated and divided. The superior stump of the vein is retracted superiorly and attached to the upper skin flap. This reflects the marginal branch away from the field of dissection. With this approach it is possible to ensure the preservation of the marginal nerve with a quick and easy maneuver that reduces the risk of damage associated with a direct identification of this thin neural structure.

Brachial Plexus

The brachial plexus emerges into the neck between the anterior and middle scalene muscles, and crosses the lower part of the posterior triangle covered by the prevertebral fascia. Injury to the brachial plexus may result in severe dysfunction of the upper limb.

Damage to the brachial plexus during neck dissection is very rare, as the plexus is protected by the prevertebral fascia. Preserving this fascia while dissecting the inferior part of the posterior triangle is crucial. However, the surgeon must be aware of the location of the brachial plexus, especially when large masses are present at this region.

6.3 General Complications

As already mentioned, poor general condition is frequently found in patients with malignant tumors of the upper aerodigestive tract undergoing functional and selective neck dissection. The incidence of associated diseases in this group of patients increases the potential for medical complications in the early postoperative period. Again, it is difficult to identify which complications can be attributed to the treatment of the primary tumor and which are the consequences of neck dissection, when both procedures are simultaneously preformed. In general, neck dissection alone, although a major head-and-neck surgical procedure, should not be regarded as a high-risk surgery, and it is not usually associated with a significant complication rate. Identification of preoperative factors that may lead to postoperative complications in this patient population not only has a predictive value but also may guide proactive interventions whenever possible.

6.3.1 Pulmonary Complications

Pulmonary complications, which are frequent after head-and-neck surgery, are probably associated with toxic habits in this group of patients. Some studies suggest increased risk of pulmonary complications with increasing exposure to smoking and drinking. However, no significant difference has been reported in the rate of pulmonary complications in patients with neck dissection. This is logical because this type of postoperative complication is very closely related to disturbance of the upper airway, which does not happen when neck dissection is performed as the sole surgical procedure.

Pneumonia and pulmonary insufficiency are the most frequent pulmonary complications after head-and-neck surgery. However, they are more closely related to the symptoms and management of the primary tumor than to neck dissection.

Pulmonary embolism is a significant cause of postoperative morbidity in general and orthopedic surgery, but it is usually not a major problem after head-and-neck surgery. Pathophysiological effects vary from small pulmonary infarcts to life-threatening cardiogenic shock. Radiological examination is required to confirm the diagnosis and to assess the extent of the problem in order to institute the most appropriate treatment. This ranges from heparin therapy to surgical embolectomy. Care of the patient with pulmonary embolism requires vigilant nursing, not only because of the risk of further embolic episodes, but also to diagnose the potential complications of treatment. Prevention of venous thromboembolism can be pharmacological or mechanical. Pulmonary embolism can occur in almost any clinical setting, but it appears most frequently in elderly, immobilized patients. Embolization rarely occurs in healthy young patients. Heart disease is the major risk factor in patients developing pulmonary embolism, with deep venous thrombosis of the legs, especially the iliac and femoral veins, as the most common precursor. Only thrombi developing in large veins are big enough to produce emboli with major clinical significance.

Pulmonary embolism usually presents with a vague clinical picture. Symptoms may be similar to those of many other cardiorespiratory disorders. Only 20% of patients show the typical symptoms—hemoptysis, pleural friction rub, gallop rhythm, cyanosis, and chest splinting. The most common physical findings are tachypnea and tachycardia, which are often transient. Arterial blood gases showing hypoxemia is nonspecific, but if arterial hypoxemia is not present, pulmonary embolism is very unlikely. There is no pathognomonic radiological sign of pulmonary embolism on the plain chest film, although cardiomegaly is the most common chest radiographic abnormality associated with acute pulmonary embolism. Reliable diagnosis depends on pulmonary arteriography, radioactive perfusion scan, or computed tomographic scan.

6.3.2 Stress Ulcer

The term *stress ulcer* refers to a heterogeneous group of acute gastric or duodenal ulcers that develop following physiologically stressful illness. Hemorrhage is the major clinical problem, although perforation occurs in about 10% of patients. Pain rarely occurs. Physical examination is not contributory except to reveal gross or occult fecal blood or signs of shock. Medication to control gastric acidity is recommended. Prophylactic treatment with inhibitors of H^+, K^+-ATPase (omeprazole, lansoprazole) are indicated in all patients undergoing neck dissection.

6.3.3 Hypoparathyroidism

Hypoparathyroidism is the most common complication after interventions in the central compartment. Damage to the parathyroid glands may be due to either deliberate or inadvertent removal of the gland, or disturbance to its vascularization. Parathyroid glands should be identified during central compartment surgery, and the specimen should be revised when some are missing, in order to reimplant those that had been removed. Most of the time, the inferior thyroid artery irrigates both the superior and the inferior parathyroid glands, although the superior thyroid artery may be the primary contributor to around 20% of superior parathyroid glands. The vascular supply to the glands should be carefully preserved during central compartment interventions, and the glands that are presumed to be poorly vascularized at the end of the surgery should be also reimplanted.

Parathyroid glands damage produces an impairment in parathyroid hormone secretion, that secondarily evolves into hypocalcemia. It is agreed that one or two functioning parathyroid glands are enough to maintain calcium homeostasis. The persistent hypocalcemia raises the resting transmembrane potential and creates a hyperexcitability status in neural and muscular cells. This results in paresthesia (typically around the mouth, and in the hands and feet), muscle cramps (tetania) and finally heart arrhythmias, bronchospasm, seizures and death.

Hypoparathyroidism is a potentially lethal complication, but symptoms don't develop for 24 to 72 hours after surgery.

A careful follow-up of the patients, including clinical and calcium monitoring, is mandatory to avoid the developing of severe hypocalcemia after discharge. Recently, several protocols have appeared to predict through pre- and/or postoperative parathyroid hormone measurements which patients can be safely discharged during the first 24 hours without the need of monitoring.

6

7 Frequently Asked Questions with Answers

Every time that we lecture about functional neck dissection, there are a number of questions that systematically appear in the discussion. In this chapter, we would like to answer these questions following the basic guidelines presented in the previous pages.

7.1 Does the Site of the Primary Tumor Influence the Type of Dissection (i.e., Functional vs. Radical)?

This question was frequently asked in the early days of functional neck dissection when the operation was not considered safe from the oncological standpoint. At that time, more aggressive neck treatment was advised for tumor sites behaving more aggressively (floor of the mouth, tongue, hypopharynx). Thus, radical neck dissection was preferred to a functional approach as a means to improve the outcome.

Nowadays we have learned to separate primary and neck. We are aware that some tumor locations have worse prognosis than others. Hypopharynx cancer is usually more aggressive than tumors of the larynx, but this will not be modified by using a different neck treatment than the one required for the clinical scenario. In other words, for an N0 neck on a patient with a piriform sinus tumor, radical neck dissection is not safer than functional neck dissection.

In head-and-neck cancer patients the neck must be treated according to its own status. The primary should not be used as a criterion for deciding the approach to the neck. The decision whether to use radical or functional neck dissection should be based only on the characteristics of the neck. However, once a functional approach has been selected, the type and extent of the dissection (complete or selective) should be determined by the location of the primary and the experience of the surgeon, as we have repeatedly emphasized in the previous pages.

7.2 Does the Number of Nodes Dictate the Type of Dissection?

This is another controversial issue concerning functional neck dissection. Again, most doubts in this respect come from the early days when functional neck dissection was considered insufficient. Although not unanimously recognized, the number of positive nodes in the neck dissection specimen may harbor prognostic information. However, the exact number of nodes defining the chances for a poor outcome varies in different studies. On the other hand, in some series, the number of nodes is not considered to be important from the prognostic standpoint. In any case, selection of the surgical approach to the neck should not be indicated by the number of nodes, but by the characteristics of every single node that has been detected in the patient's neck.

Functional neck dissection can be performed in patients with nonpalpable and small palpable mobile nodes (usually smaller than 2.5 cm), the size being just a merely orienting factor. The operation is totally safe in patients with multiple nodes, as long as all nodes fulfill these criteria. In these cases, radical neck dissection will not be safer than a functional approach. Thus, it is not the number of nodes that is important, but their clinical characteristics.

7.3 Do You Always Use Postoperative Radiation Therapy after Functional Neck Dissection in $_pN$ + Patients?

We would very much like to have a conclusive answer to the question of postoperative radiotherapy for positive nodes, but unfortunately this is not the case. In fact, nobody has the answer to this question.

Postoperative radiotherapy has been recommended in a large variety of situations: for all patients with positive nodes; only for patients with more than a certain number of positive nodes—the number being as variable as the authors that propose this approach; only for patients with positive nodes showing extracapsular extension; and also, for a number of combinations of the above.

In our experience, postoperative radiotherapy does not improve regional control or survival in previously untreated patients with cancer of the larynx undergoing surgical treatment—all patients in this series had functional neck dissection as part of the initial treatment. Several aspects of the previous statement should be emphasized: (1) This series includes only patients with cancer of the larynx, a special subset of head-and-neck cancer patients with particular characteristics. Extension of this statement to other tumor locations requires further studies. (2) Patients included in this study were N0 patients with occult disease and patients with palpable mobile nodes smaller than 2.5 cm. (3) All patients in our series were treated with the same functional approach, removing all lymph node regions except level I. (4) The study was performed retrospectively with a historical control from the same institution. Although this may be considered a weak point of the study, it must be remembered that the great majority of studies trying to assess the usefulness of postoperative radiotherapy are retrospective studies.

7

With this in mind, we can affirm that postoperative radiotherapy did not improve the outcome of our patients (survival and regional control) in any situation. Patients with positive nodes did worse than those without nodes; and patients with extracapsular spread had an especially bad prognosis. However, this was not improved or modified by the addition of postoperative radiotherapy.

In conclusion, we do not routinely use postoperative radiotherapy in pN+ patients with cancer of the larynx treated with functional neck dissection. In contrast to "routine use," we encourage an individualized approach to cancer patient management, evaluating all variables and selecting the best option for every single patient. We do not believe there is a "treatment of choice," but rather consider that we have "choices of treatment" and try to fit the treatment to the patient and not the patient to the treatment.

7.4 Is Functional Neck Dissection Still Possible in Previously Irradiated Patients?

This is a philosophical rather than a technical issue. Functional neck dissection is based on fascial compartmentalization of the neck. The fascial spaces of the neck separate the lymphatic tissue from the remaining neck structures. As a consequence of this definition, functional neck dissection is not possible in a previously irradiated patient because destruction of the fascial spaces within the neck is one of the unavoidable consequences of radiation therapy. Thus, fascial neck dissection is not possible after radiation to the neck.

According to the clinical scenario, some type of nonradical neck dissection may be possible in previously irradiated patients. However, these operations are not true functional neck dissections but technical modifications to radical neck dissection in which emphasis is placed on preserving selected neck structures not involved by the tumor. These are "modified radical neck dissections," operations based on the principles described by Crile, in which some preservation is attempted.

This situation clearly illustrates the conceptual difference between the *functional* and the *classic* approach to neck dissection.

7.5 May Functional Neck Dissection Be Used as a Salvage Operation for Treatment Failures?

The same answer can be given to this question. Previous surgery modifies the fascial planes of the neck, thus making functional neck dissection not possible. Again, some structures not involved by the tumor may be preserved at surgery. However, this will not be a true functional approach but a modified radical neck dissection.

7.6 Is Functional Neck Dissection Still Possible after Open Nodal Biopsy?

In most cases, no functional approach is possible after a previous open biopsy of the neck. An open nodal biopsy usually impedes a functional approach to the neck.

The discussion about the drawbacks of open nodal biopsy started more than 60 years ago, during the time of Hayes Martin. Later studies supported that open neck biopsy was harmful in terms of increased wound necrosis, cervical recurrence, and distant metastasis. However, subsequent studies suggested that there is no detriment to survival or recurrence if definitive treatment follows the biopsy without significant delay. A significant detriment to the patient after open neck biopsy is that more structures need to be sacrificed at the time of definitive neck surgery, because a functional approach will not be possible after open nodal biopsy. At present, this is one of the most important arguments against open neck biopsy.

7.7 How Do You Approach a Patient with Small Bilateral Nodes Suitable for Bilateral Functional Neck Dissection?

A frequent concern in bilateral neck dissection when both sides of the neck are clinically positive is whether it will be possible to preserve at least one internal jugular vein.

In some instances, this may be solved by starting the dissection on the "good" side—the one with smaller nodes. This will probably ensure the preservation of the internal jugular vein on the first side, allowing a more aggressive approach on the "bad" side. However, this approach may prove impractical if the internal jugular vein is injured or must be sacrificed on the good side. In such instances the dissection of the opposite, or bad, side may be delayed approximately 3 weeks, or may be performed, accepting the risk associated with the simultaneous removal of both internal jugular veins. The final decision depends more on surgeons' preferences than on patient characteristics.

7.8 When Bilateral Functional Neck Dissection Is Indicated and the Internal Jugular Vein Is Damaged during the Dissection of the First Side, Will You Continue the Operation, or Do You Prefer to Stage the Second Side?

The easiest answer is: do not damage the internal jugular vein during surgery. However, this is not always possible and accidents do happen. On the other hand, sometimes the vein must be sacrificed on one side for oncological reasons. In such circumstances we will probably continue the operation and dissect the opposite side if the clinical situation suggests a reasonable chance of preserving the contralateral vein. The chances of accidental damage to the opposite internal jugular vein are low and there is a high probability that the operation can be completed in a single surgical time without problems.

The situation is different if radical neck dissection is planned on the opposite side or the chances to preserve the opposite internal jugular vein are low. Here the decision is more difficult. Staging the operation means not operating the side with the higher stage of disease and waiting approximately 3 weeks before definitive treatment may be accomplished. This should be regarded as potentially harmful for the patient. The alternative is to continue the operation, trying to preserve as much superficial venous drainage as possible, keeping in mind that oncological safety is much more important than venous preservation. When no superficial drainage can be preserved and both internal jugular veins are removed in the same operation, the patient must be carefully managed in the intensive care unit, and appropriate hydroelectrolytic balance should be maintained. In spite of these maneuvers, there is a high risk of severe complications. Thus, the final decision should be taken according to the patient status and clinical scenario.

7.9 Which Is Your Approach to Borderline Indications: Functional or Radical?

Dealing with borderline indications requires clear concepts to avoid faulty decisions. There are two basic oncological premises that must guide the surgeon's mind when facing a borderline case:

1. Life is more important than function.
2. The first treatment is the most likely to succeed.

With this in mind the surgeon must decide the most appropriate approach for every single case. Most of the time this will probably be a more aggressive approach than desired. It must be clear to every head-and-neck surgeon that cancer cells cannot be "chased" with a knife, and technical demonstrations of surgical expertise are not good for the patient and should be limited to the dissection room.

In conclusion, when in doubt, choose the procedure that, in your own personal experience, offers the patient the highest chance for cure. Establishing priorities is one of the first things that every surgeon must learn, and for head-and-neck cancer surgery life is the first priority to consider.

7.10 What Will You Do with a Lymph Node Contacting the Internal Jugular Vein?

The situation is similar to that presented in the previous question. Thus, the answer should be the same.

There is no need to look for—or even worse, create—a cleavage plane between the internal jugular vein and an adjacent lymph node in order to separate the node from the vein and preserve the latter. After all, the internal jugular vein is just "a vein with a name." There is almost no morbidity associated with the removal of one internal jugular vein, and there may be important disadvantages from an oncological standpoint if the limits are pushed too far. Thus, in case of doubt we strongly recommend the removal of the internal jugular vein, or any other removable structure adjacent to a metastatic lymph node, if this may increase the chances for cure.

The situation is more difficult when the internal jugular vein has been sacrificed, or must also be removed, on the opposite side. In these cases, the advantages and disadvantages of preserving the vein on the "good" side and performing a one-stage operation must be weighed against those associated with a two-stage procedure in which the second side is operated approximately 3 weeks later, and also against those derived from a simultaneous bilateral removal of the internal jugular vein. Here, the clinical scenario and the surgeon's experience are crucial to selecting the most appropriate decision for every patient.

7

Suggested Readings

[1] Acar A, Dursun G, Aydin O, Akbaş Y. J incision in neck dissections. J Laryngol Otol. ; 112(1):55–60

[2] AJCC. Cancer Staging Manual. 8th ed. Springer International Publishing; 2017

[3] Al-Sarraf M, Pajak TF, Byhardt RW, Beitler JJ, Salter MM, Cooper JS. Postoperative radiotherapy with concurrent cisplatin appears to improve locoregional control of advanced, resectable head and neck cancers: RTOG 88-24. Int J Radiat Oncol Biol Phys. ; 37(4):777–782

[4] Carty SE, Cooper DS, Doherty GM, et al. American Thyroid Association Surgery Working Group, American Association of Endocrine Surgeons, American Academy of Otolaryngology-Head and Neck Surgery, American Head and Neck Society. Consensus statement on the terminology and classification of central neck dissection for thyroid cancer. Thyroid. ; 19(11): 1153–1158

[5] Andersen PE, Cambronero E, Shaha AR, Shah JP. The extent of neck disease after regional failure during observation of the N0 neck. Am J Surg. ; 172(6): 689–691

[6] Andersen PE, Shah JP, Cambronero E, Spiro RH. The role of comprehensive neck dissection with preservation of the spinal accessory nerve in the clinically positive neck. Am J Surg. ; 168(5):499–502

[7] Ariyan S. Functional radical neck dissection. Plast Reconstr Surg. ; 65(6): 768–776

[8] Armstrong J, Pfister D, Strong E, et al. The management of the clinically positive neck as part of a larynx preservation approach. Int J Radiat Oncol Biol Phys. ; 26(5):759–765

[9] Arriaga MA, Kanel KT, Johnson JT, Myers EN. Medical complications in total laryngectomy: incidence and risk factors. Ann Otol Rhinol Laryngol. ; 99(8): 611–615

[10] Avalos E, Beltrán M, Martín A, et al. Factores de predicción de la invasión ganglionar en el carcinoma de laringe. Acta Otorrinolaringol Esp. ; 49(6): 452–454

[11] Bailey BJ. Selective neck dissection: the challenge of occult metastases. Arch Otolaryngol Head Neck Surg. ; 124(3):353

[12] Ballantyne AJ, Jackson GL. Synchronous bilateral neck dissection. Am J Surg. ; 144(4):452–455

[13] Banerjee AR, Alun-Jones T. Neck dissection. Clin Otolaryngol Allied Sci. ; 20 (4):286–290

[14] Bartelink H, Breur K, Hart G, Annyas B, van Slooten E, Snow G. The value of postoperative radiotherapy as an adjuvant to radical neck dissection. Cancer. ; 52(6):1008–1013

[15] Barzan L, Talamini R. Analysis of prognostic factors for recurrence after neck dissection. Arch Otolaryngol Head Neck Surg. ; 122(12):1299–1302

[16] Beenken SW, Krontiras H, Maddox WA, Peters GE, Soong S, Urist MM. T1 and T2 squamous cell carcinoma of the oral tongue: prognostic factors and the role of elective lymph node dissection. Head Neck. ; 21(2):124–130

[17] Betka J, Mrzena L, Astl J, et al. Surgical treatment strategy for thyroid gland carcinoma nodal metastases. Eur Arch Otorhinolaryngol. ; 254 Suppl 1: S169–S174

[18] Bhattacharyya N. The effects of more conservative neck dissections and radiotherapy on nodal yields from the neck. Arch Otolaryngol Head Neck Surg. ; 124(4):412–416

[19] Bocca E, Pignataro O, Oldini C, Cappa C. Functional neck dissection: an evaluation and review of 843 cases. Laryngoscope. ; 94(7):942–945

[20] Bocca E, Pignataro O, Sasaki CT. Functional neck dissection. A description of operative technique. Arch Otolaryngol. ; 106(9):524–527

[21] Bocca E, Pignataro O. A conservation technique in radical neck dissection. Ann Otol Rhinol Laryngol. ; 76(5):975–987

[22] Bocca E. Conservative neck dissection. Laryngoscope. ; 85(9):1511–1515

[23] Bocca E. Functional problems connected with bilateral radical neck dissection. J Laryngol Otol. ; 67(9):567–577

[24] Bocca E. Supraglottic laryngectomy and functional neck dissection. J Laryngol Otol. ; 80(8):831–838

[25] Bonner JA, Harari PM, Giralt J, et al. Radiotherapy plus cetuximab for squamous-cell carcinoma of the head and neck. N Engl J Med. ; 354(6):567–578

[26] Breau RL, Suen JY. Management of the N(0) neck. Otolaryngol Clin North Am. ; 31(4):657–669

[27] Brown DH, Mulholland S, Yoo JH, et al. Internal jugular vein thrombosis following modified neck dissection: implications for head and neck flap reconstruction. Head Neck. ; 20(2):169–174

[28] Brown JJ, Fee WE, Jr. Management of the neck in nasopharyngeal carcinoma (NPC). Otolaryngol Clin North Am. ; 31(5):785–802

[29] Byers RM, Clayman GL, McGill D, et al. Selective neck dissections for squamous carcinoma of the upper aerodigestive tract: patterns of regional failure. Head Neck. ; 21(6):499–505

[30] Byers RM, El-Naggar AK, Lee YY, et al. Can we detect or predict the presence of occult nodal metastases in patients with squamous carcinoma of the oral tongue? Head Neck. ; 20(2):138–144

[31] Byers RM, Wolf PF, Ballantyne AJ. Rationale for elective modified neck dissection. Head Neck Surg. ; 10(3):160–167

[32] Byers RM. Modified neck dissection. A study of 967 cases from 1970 to 1980. Am J Surg. ; 150(4):414–421

[33] Byers RM. Neck dissection: concepts, controversies, and technique. Semin Surg Oncol. ; 7(1):9–13

[34] Cabra J, Herranz J, Moñux A, Gavilán J. Postoperative complications after functional neck dissection. Oper Tech Otolaryngol–Head Neck Surg. ; 4:318–321

[35] Calearo CV, Teatini G. Functional neck dissection. Anatomical grounds, surgical technique, clinical observations. Ann Otol Rhinol Laryngol. ; 92(3, Pt 1):215–222

[36] Califano J, Westra WH, Koch W, et al. Unknown primary head and neck squamous cell carcinoma: molecular identification of the site of origin. J Natl Cancer Inst. ; 91(7):599–604

[37] Califano L, Zupi A, Mangone GM, Longo F, Coscia G, Piombino P. Surgical management of the neck in squamous cell carcinoma of the tongue. Br J Oral Maxillofac Surg. ; 37(4):320–323

[38] Candela FC, Kothari K, Shah JP. Patterns of cervical node metastases from squamous carcinoma of the oropharynx and hypopharynx. Head Neck. ; 12 (3):197–203

[39] Carter RL. The pathologist's appraisal of neck dissections. Eur Arch Otorhinolaryngol. ; 250(8):429–431

[40] Cheng PT, Hao SP, Lin YH, Yeh AR. Objective comparison of shoulder dysfunction after three neck dissection techniques. Ann Otol Rhinol Laryngol. ; 109(8, Pt 1):761–766

[41] Chu W, Strawitz JG. Results in suprahyoid, modified radical, and standard radical neck dissections for metastatic squamous cell carcinoma: recurrence and survival. Am J Surg. ; 136(4):512–515

[42] Clark JR, Busse PM, Norris CM, Jr, et al. Induction chemotherapy with cisplatin, fluorouracil, and high-dose leucovorin for squamous cell carcinoma of the head and neck: long-term results. J Clin Oncol. ; 15(9): 3100–3110

[43] Clayman GL, Eicher SA, Sicard MW, Razmpa E, Goepfert H. Surgical outcomes in head and neck cancer patients 80 years of age and older. Head Neck. ; 20(3):216–223

[44] Clayman GL, Frank DK. Selective neck dissection of anatomically appropriate levels is as efficacious as modified radical neck dissection for elective treatment of the clinically negatice neck in patients with squamous cell carcinoma of the upper respiratory and digestive tracts. Arch Otolaryngol Head Neck Surg. ; 124(3):348–352

[45] Close LG, Burns DK, Reisch J, Schaefer SD. Microvascular invasion in cancer of the oral cavity and oropharynx. Arch Otolaryngol Head Neck Surg. ; 113 (11):1191–1195

[46] Cohen L. Theoretical "iso-survival" formulae for fractionated radiation therapy. Br J Radiol. ; 41(487):522–528

[47] Conley J. The management of metastatic cancer in the region of the head and neck. Minn Med. ; 50(6):992

[48] Cousins VC, Milton CM, Bickerton RC. Hospital morbidity and mortality following total laryngectomy. Experience of 374 operations. J Laryngol Otol. ; 101(11):1159–1164

[49] Coutard H. Roentgentherapy of epitheliomas of the tonsilar region, hypopharynx and larynx from 1920 to 1926. Am J Roent. ; 28:313–343

[50] Crile G. Excision of cancer of the head and neck with special reference to the plan of dissection based on 132 operations. JAMA. ; 47:1780–1785

[51] Danninger R, Posawetz W, Humer U, Stammberger H, Jakse R. [Ultrasound investigation of cervical lymph node metastases: conception and results of a histopathological exploration]. Laryngorhinootologie. ; 78(3):144–149

[52] Davidson BJ, Kulkarny V, Delacure MD, Shah JP. Posterior triangle metastases of squamous cell carcinoma of the upper aerodigestive tract. Am J Surg. ; 166(4):395–398

7

[53] Davidson J, Khan Y, Gilbert R, Birt BD, Balogh J, MacKenzie R. Is selective neck dissection sufficient treatment for the N0/Np+neck? J Otolaryngol. ; 26(4):229–231

[54] de Campora E, Radici M, Camaioni A, Pianelli C. Clinical experiences with surgical therapy of cervical metastases from head and neck cancer. Eur Arch Otorhinolaryngol. ; 251(6):335–341

[55] de Gier HH, Balm AJ, Bruning PF, Gregor RT, Hilgers FJ. Systematic approach to the treatment of chylous leakage after neck dissection. Head Neck. ; 18 (4):347–351

[56] Decker DA, Drelichman A, Jacobs J, et al. Adjuvant chemotherapy with cis-diamminodichloroplatinum II and 120-hour infusion 5-fluorouracil in Stage III and IV squamous cell carcinoma of the head and neck. Cancer. ; 51(8):1353–1355

[57] Del Sel JA, Agra A. Cancer of the larynx: laryngectomy with systemic extirpation of the connective tissue and cervical lymph nodes as a routine procedure. Trans Am Acad Ophthalmol Otolaryngol. ; 51:653–655

[58] Wolf GT, Fisher SG, Hong WK, et al. Department of Veterans Affairs Laryngeal Cancer Study Group. Induction chemotherapy plus radiation compared with surgery plus radiation in patients with advanced laryngeal cancer. N Engl J Med. ; 324(24):1685–1690

[59] DeSanto LW, Beahrs OH, Holt JJ, O'Fallon WM. Neck dissection and combined therapy. Study of effectiveness. Arch Otolaryngol. ; 111(6):366–370

[60] DeSanto LW, Beahrs OH. Modified and complete neck dissection in the treatment of squamous cell carcinoma of the head and neck. Surg Gynecol Obstet. ; 167(3):259–269

[61] DeSanto LW, Holt JJ, Beahrs OH, O'Fallon WM. Neck dissection: is it worthwhile? Laryngoscope. ; 92(5):502–509

[62] Dulguerov P, Soulier C, Maurice J, Faidutti B, Allal AS, Lehmann W. Bilateral radical neck dissection with unilateral internal jugular vein reconstruction. Laryngoscope. ; 108(11, Pt 1):1692–1696

[63] Elliott CG, Goldhaber SZ, Visani L, DeRosa M. Chest radiographs in acute pulmonary embolism. Results from the International Cooperative Pulmonary Embolism Registry. Chest. ; 118(1):33–38

[64] Enepekides DJ, Sultanem K, Nguyen C, Shenouda G, Black MJ, Rochon L. Occult cervical metastases: immunoperoxidase analysis of the pathologically negative neck. Otolaryngol Head Neck Surg. ; 120(5):713–717

[65] Ensley JF, Jacobs JR, Weaver A, et al. Correlation between response to cisplatinum-combination chemotherapy and subsequent radiotherapy in previously untreated patients with advanced squamous cell cancers of the head and neck. Cancer. ; 54(5):811–814

[66] Fagan JJ, Collins B, Barnes L, D'Amico F, Myers EN, Johnson JT. Perineural invasion in squamous cell carcinoma of the head and neck. Arch Otolaryngol Head Neck Surg. ; 124(6):637–640

[67] Farrar WB, Finkelmeier WR, McCabe DP, Young DC, O'Dwyer PJ, James AG. Radical neck dissection: is it enough? Am J Surg. ; 156(3, Pt 1):173–176

[68] Feinmesser R, Freeman JL, Noyek AM, Birt BD. Metastatic neck disease. A clinical/radiographic/pathologic correlative study. Arch Otolaryngol Head Neck Surg. ; 113(12):1307–1310

[69] Ferlito A, Rinaldo A. Level I dissection for laryngeal and hypopharyngeal cancer: is it indicated? J Laryngol Otol. ; 112(5):438–440

[70] Ferlito A, Rinaldo A. Selective lateral neck dissection for laryngeal cancer in the clinically negative neck: is it justified? J Laryngol Otol. ; 112(10):921–924

[71] Ferlito A, Rinaldo A. Selective lateral neck dissection for laryngeal cancer with limited metastatic disease: is it indicated? J Laryngol Otol. ; 112(11):1031–1033

[72] Ferlito A, Robbins KT, Shah JP, et al. Proposal for a rational classification of neck dissections. Head Neck. ; 33(3):445–450

[73] Ferlito A, Silver CE, Rinaldo A, Smith RV. Surgical treatment of the neck in cancer of the larynx. ORL J Otorhinolaryngol Relat Spec. ; 62(4):217–225

[74] Ferlito A, Som PM, Rinaldo A, Mondin V. Classification and terminology of neck dissections. ORL J Otorhinolaryngol Relat Spec. ; 62(4):212–216

[75] Fisch UP, Sigel ME. Cervical lymphatic system as visualized by lymphography. Ann Otol Rhinol Laryngol. ; 73:870–882

[76] Fletcher GH, Shukovsky LJ. The interplay of radiocurability and tolerance in the irradiation of human cancers. J Radiol Electrol Med Nucl. ; 56(5):383–400

[77] Fletcher GH. Clinical dose-response curves of human malignant epithelial tumours. Br J Radiol. ; 46(541):1–12

[78] Fletcher GH. Elective irradiation of subclinical disease in cancers of the head and neck. Cancer. ; 29(6):1450–1454

[79] Forastiere AA, Goepfert H, Maor M, et al. Concurrent chemotherapy and radiotherapy for organ preservation in advanced laryngeal cancer. N Engl J Med. ; 349(22):2091–2098

[80] Forastiere AA, Maor M, Weber RS, et al. Long-term results of Intergroup RTOG 91–11: a phase III trial to preserve the larynx–Induction cisplatin/5-FU and radiation therapy versus concurrent cisplatin and radiation therapy versus radiation therapy. ASCO Meeting Abstracts 2006;24(18, Suppl):5517

[81] Friedman M, Lim JW, Dickey W, et al. Quantification of lymph nodes in selective neck dissection. Laryngoscope. ; 109(3):368–370

[82] Friedman M, Mafee MF, Pacella BL, Jr, Strorigl TL, Dew LL, Toriumi DM. Rationale for elective neck dissection in 1990. Laryngoscope. ; 100(1):54–59

[83] Fulciniti F, Califano L, Zupi A, Vetrani A. Accuracy of fine needle aspiration biopsy in head and neck tumors. J Oral Maxillofac Surg. ; 55(10):1094–1097

[84] Gavilán Alonso C, Blanco Galdín A, Suárez Nieto C. El vaciamiento funcional-radical cervicoganglionar. Anatomía quirúrgica. Técnica y resultados. Acta Otorinolaringol Iber Am. ; 23(5):703–817

[85] Gavilán J, Gavilán C, Herranz J. Functional neck dissection: three decades of controversy. Ann Otol Rhinol Laryngol. ; 101(4):339–341

[86] Gavilán J, Gavilán C, Mañós-Pujol M, Herranz J. Discriminant analysis in predicting survival of patients with cancer of the larynx or hypopharynx. Clin Otolaryngol Allied Sci. ; 12(5):331–335

[87] Gavilán C, Gavilán J. Five-year results of functional neck dissection for cancer of the larynx. Arch Otolaryngol Head Neck Surg. ; 115(10):1193–1196

[88] Gavilán J, Moñux A, Herranz J, Gavilán C. Functional neck dissection: surgical technique. Oper Tech Otolaryngol–Head Neck Surg. ; 4:258–265

[89] Gavilán J, Prim MP, De Diego JI, Hardisson D, Pozuelo A. Postoperative radiotherapy in patients with positive nodes after functional neck dissection. Ann Otol Rhinol Laryngol. ; 109(9):844–848

[90] Giacomarra V, Tirelli G, Papanikolla L, Bussani R. Predictive factors of nodal metastases in oral cavity and oropharynx carcinomas. Laryngoscope. ; 109 (5):795–799

[91] Gillies EM, Luna MA. Histologic evaluation of neck dissection specimens. Otolaryngol Clin North Am. ; 31(5):759–771

[92] Goepfert H, Jesse RH, Ballantyne AJ. Posterolateral neck dissection. Arch Otolaryngol. ; 106(10):618–620

[93] Goodwin WJ, Jr, Chandler JR. Indications for radical neck dissection following radiation therapy. Arch Otolaryngol. ; 104(7):367–370

[94] Grandi C, Alloisio M, Moglia D, et al. Prognostic significance of lymphatic spread in head and neck carcinomas: therapeutic implications. Head Neck Surg. ; 8(2):67–73

[95] Güney E, Yiğitbaşi OG, Canöz K, Oztürk M, Ersoy A. Functional neck dissection: cure and functional results. J Laryngol Otol. ; 112(12):1176–1178

[96] Güney E, Yigitbasi OG. Management of N0 neck in T1-T2 unilateral supraglottic cancer. Ann Otol Rhinol Laryngol. ; 108(10):998–1003

[97] Haddadin KJ, Soutar DS, Oliver RJ, Webster MH, Robertson AG, MacDonald DG. Improved survival for patients with clinically T1/T2, N0 tongue tumors undergoing a prophylactic neck dissection. Head Neck. ; 21(6):517–525

[98] Haller JR, Mountain RE, Schuller DE, Nag S. Mortality and morbidity with intraoperative radiotherapy for head and neck cancer. Am J Otolaryngol. ; 17 (5):308–310

[99] Henick DH, Silver CE, Heller KS, Shaha AR, El GH, Wolk DP. Supraomohyoid neck dissection as a staging procedure for squamous cell carcinomas of the oral cavity and oropharynx. Head Neck. ; 17(2):119–123

[100] Herranz J, Sarandeses A, Fernández MF, Barro CV, Vidal JM, Gavilán J. Complications after total laryngectomy in nonradiated laryngeal and hypopharyngeal carcinomas. Otolaryngol Head Neck Surg. ; 122(6):892–898

[101] Hillel AD. Disability resulting from radical and modified neck dissections. Head Neck Surg. ; 9(2):127–129

[102] Hoffman HT, Porter K, Karnell LH, et al. Laryngeal cancer in the United States: changes in demographics, patterns of care, and survival. Laryngoscope. ; 116(9, Pt 2) Suppl 111:1–13

[103] Hollinshead WH. Anatomy for Surgeons: The Head and Neck. 3rd ed. Philadelphia, PA: JB Lippincott; 1982

[104] Jesse RH, Ballantyne AJ, Larson D. Radical or modified neck dissection: a therapeutic dilemma. Am J Surg. ; 136(4):516–519

[105] Jesse RH, Barkley HT, Jr, Lindberg RD, Fletcher GH. Cancer of the oral cavity. Is elective neck dissection beneficial? Am J Surg. ; 120(4):505–508

[106] Jesse RH, Fletcher GH. Treatment of the neck in patients with squamous cell carcinoma of the head and neck. Cancer. ; 39(2) Suppl:868–872

[107] Jesse RH, Lindberg RD. The efficacy of combining radiation therapy with a surgical procedure in patients with cervical metastasis from squamous cancer of the oropharynx and hypopharynx. Cancer. ; 35(4):1163–1166

7

[108] Johnson CR, Silverman LN, Clay LB, Schmidt-Ullrich R. Radiotherapeutic management of bulky cervical lymphadenopathy in squamous cell carcinoma of the head and neck: is postradiotherapy neck dissection necessary? Radiat Oncol Investig. ; 6(1):52–57

[109] Johnson JT, Barnes EL, Myers EN, Schramm VL, Jr, Borochovitz D, Sigler BA. The extracapsular spread of tumors in cervical node metastasis. Arch Otolaryngol. ; 107(12):725–729

[110] Johnson JT, Kachman K, Wagner RL, Myers EN. Comparison of ampicillin/sulbactam versus clindamycin in the prevention of infection in patients undergoing head and neck surgery. Head Neck. ; 19(5):367–371

[111] Johnson JT, Myers EN, Bedetti CD, Barnes EL, Schramm VL, Jr, Thearle PB. Cervical lymph node metastases. Incidence and implications of extracapsular carcinoma. Arch Otolaryngol. ; 111(8):534–537

[112] Johnson JT. Selective neck dissection in patients with squamous cell carcinoma of the upper respiratory and digestive tracts: a lack of adequate data. Arch Otolaryngol Head Neck Surg. ; 124(3):353

[113] Jones TA, Stell PM. The preservation of shoulder function after radical neck dissection. Clin Otolaryngol Allied Sci. ; 10(2):89–92

[114] Joseph CA, Gregor RT, Davidge-Pitts KJ. The role of functional neck dissection in the management of advanced tumours of the upper aerodigestive tract. S Afr J Surg. ; 23(3):83–87

[115] Kaufman R, Strauss M. Conservation surgery of the neck: modified neck dissection. Trans Pa Acad Ophthalmol Otolaryngol. ; 35(1):43–47

[116] Kerrebijn JD, Freeman JL, Irish JC, et al. Supraomohyoid neck dissection. Is it diagnostic or therapeutic? Head Neck. ; 21(1):39–42

[117] Koch WM, Choti MA, Civelek AC, Eisele DW, Saunders JR. Gamma probe-directed biopsy of the sentinel node in oral squamous cell carcinoma. Arch Otolaryngol Head Neck Surg. ; 124(4):455–459

[118] Kowalski LP, Bagietto R, Lara JR, Santos RL, Tagawa EK, Santos IR. Factors influencing contralateral lymph node metastasis from oral carcinoma. Head Neck. ; 21(2):104–110

[119] Kowalski LP, Magrin J, Waksman G, et al. Supraomohyoid neck dissection in the treatment of head and neck tumors. Survival results in 212 cases. Arch Otolaryngol Head Neck Surg. ; 119(9):958–963

[120] Kowalski LP, Medina JE. Nodal metastases: predictive factors. Otolaryngol Clin North Am. ; 31(4):621–637

[121] Köybasioglu A, Tokcaer AB, Uslu S, Ileri F, Beder L, Ozbilen S. Accessory nerve function after modified radical and lateral neck dissections. Laryngoscope. ; 110(1):73–77

[122] Kramer S, Gelber RD, Snow JB, et al. Combined radiation therapy and surgery in the management of advanced head and neck cancer: final report of study 73–03 of the Radiation Therapy Oncology Group. Head Neck Surg. ; 10(1):19–30

[123] Kraus DH, Carew JF, Harrison LB. Regional lymph node metastasis from cutaneous squamous cell carcinoma. Arch Otolaryngol Head Neck Surg. ; 124(5):582–587

[124] Kuntz AL, Weymuller EA, Jr. Impact of neck dissection on quality of life. Laryngoscope. ; 109(8):1334–1338

[125] Lawrence W, Jr, Terz JJ, Rogers C, King RE, Wolf JS, King ER. Proceedings: preoperative irradiation for head and neck cancer: a prospective study. Cancer. ; 33(2):318–323

[126] Leemans CR, Snow GB. Is selective neck dissection really as efficacious as modified radical neck dissection for elective treatment of the clinically negative neck in patients with squamous cell carcinoma of the upper respiratory and digestive tracts? Arch Otolaryngol Head Neck Surg. ; 124(9):1042–1044

[127] Leemans CR, Tiwari R, van der Waal I, Karim AB, Nauta JJ, Snow GB. The efficacy of comprehensive neck dissection with or without postoperative radiotherapy in nodal metastases of squamous cell carcinoma of the upper respiratory and digestive tracts. Laryngoscope. ; 100(11):1194–1198

[128] Lefebvre JL, Chevalier D, Luboinski B, Kirkpatrick A, Collette L, Sahmoud T, EORTC Head and Neck Cancer Cooperative Group. Larynx preservation in pyriform sinus cancer: preliminary results of a European Organization for Research and Treatment of Cancer phase III trial. J Natl Cancer Inst. ; 88(13):890–899

[129] Leipzig B, Suen JY, English JL, Barnes J, Hooper M. Functional evaluation of the spinal accessory nerve after neck dissection. Am J Surg. ; 146(4):526–530

[130] Levendag P, Sessions R, Vikram B, et al. The problem of neck relapse in early stage supraglottic larynx cancer. Cancer. ; 63(2):345–348

[131] Levertu P, Adelstein DJ, Saxton JP, et al. Management of the neck in a randomized trial comparing concurrent chemotherapy and radiation with radiotherapy alone in resectable stage III and IV squamous cell carcinoma. Head Neck Surg. ; 19:559–566

[132] Lavertu P, Bonafede JP, Adelstein DJ, et al. Comparison of surgical complications after organ-preservation therapy in patients with stage III or IV squamous cell head and neck cancer. Arch Otolaryngol Head Neck Surg. ; 124(4):401–406

[133] Lindberg R. Distribution of cervical lymph node metastases from squamous cell carcinoma of the upper respiratory and digestive tracts. Cancer. ; 29(6):1446–1449

[134] Lingeman RE, Helmus C, Stephens R, Ulm J. Neck dissection: radical or conservative. Ann Otol Rhinol Laryngol. ; 86(6, Pt 1):737–744

[135] Lundahl RE, Foote RL, Bonner JA, et al. Combined neck dissection and postoperative radiation therapy in the management of the high-risk neck: a matched-pair analysis. Int J Radiat Oncol Biol Phys. ; 40(3):529–534

[136] Lydiatt DD, Karrer FW, Lydiatt WM, Johnson PJ. The evaluation, indications, and contraindications of selective neck dissections. Nebr Med J. ; 79(5):140–144

[137] Lyons AJ, Mills CC. Anatomical variants of the cervical sympathetic chain to be considered during neck dissection. Br J Oral Maxillofac Surg. ; 36(3):180–182

[138] Mabanta SR, Mendenhall WM, Stringer SP, Cassisi NJ. Salvage treatment for neck recurrence after irradiation alone for head and neck squamous cell carcinoma with clinically positive neck nodes. Head Neck. ; 21(7):591–594

[139] MacComb WS, Fletcher GH. Planned combination of surgery and radiation in treatment of advanced primary head and neck cancers. Am J Roentgenol Radium Ther Nucl Med. ; 77(3):397–414

[140] Machtay M, Moughan J, Trotti A, et al. Factors associated with severe late toxicity after concurrent chemoradiation for locally advanced head and neck cancer: an RTOG analysis. J Clin Oncol. ; 26(21):3582–3589

[141] Magnano M, De Stefani A, Lerda W, et al. Prognostic factors of cervical lymph node metastasis in head and neck squamous cell carcinoma. Tumori. ; 83(6):922–926

[142] Mahasin ZZ, Saleem M, Gangopadhyay K. Transverse sinus thrombosis and venous infarction of the brain following unilateral radical neck dissection. J Laryngol Otol. ; 112(1):88–91

[143] Majoufre C, Faucher A, Laroche C, et al. Supraomohyoid neck dissection in cancer of the oral cavity. Am J Surg. ; 178(1):73–77

[144] Mamelle G, Pampurik J, Luboinski B, Lancar R, Lusinchi A, Bosq J. Lymph node prognostic factors in head and neck squamous cell carcinomas. Am J Surg. ; 168(5):494–498

[145] Mann W, Wolfensberger M, Füller U, Beck C. [Radical versus modified neck dissection. Cancer-related and functional viewpoints]. Laryngorhinootologie. ; 70(1):32–35

[146] Manni JJ, van den Hoogen FJ. Supraomohyoid neck dissection with frozen section biopsy as a staging procedure in the clinically node-negative neck in carcinoma of the oral cavity. Am J Surg. ; 162(4):373–376

[147] Manning M, Stell PM. The shoulder after radical neck dissection. Clin Otolaryngol Allied Sci. ; 14(5):381–384

[148] Martin H, Del Valle B, Ehrlich H, Cahan WG. Neck dissection. Cancer. ; 4(3):441–499

[149] Matsumoto M, Komiyama K, Okaue M, et al. Predicting tumor metastasis in patients with oral cancer by means of the proliferation marker Ki67. J Oral Sci. ; 41(2):53–56

[150] McCulloch TM, Jensen NF, Girod DA, Tsue TT, Weymuller EA, Jr. Risk factors for pulmonary complications in the postoperative head and neck surgery patient. Head Neck. ; 19(5):372–377

[151] McGuirt WF, Jr, Johnson JT, Myers EN, Rothfield R, Wagner R. Floor of mouth carcinoma. The management of the clinically negative neck. Arch Otolaryngol Head Neck Surg. ; 121(3):278–282

[152] McQuarrie DG, Mayberg M, Ferguson M, Shons AR. A physiologic approach to the problems of simultaneous bilateral neck dissection. Am J Surg. ; 134(4):455–460

[153] Medina JE, Byers RM. Supraomohyoid neck dissection: rationale, indications, and surgical technique. Head Neck. ; 11(2):111–122

[154] Medina JE. A rational classification of neck dissections. Otolaryngol Head Neck Surg. ; 100(3):169–176

[155] Medina JE. Neck dissection in the treatment of cancer of major salivary glands. Otolaryngol Clin North Am. ; 31(5):815–822

[156] Montgomery RL. Head and Neck Anatomy with Clinical Correlations. New York: McGraw-Hill; 1981

[157] Moore KL. Clinically Oriented Anatomy. 3rd ed. Baltimore, MD: Williams & Wilkins; 1992

7

[158] Moreau A, Goffart Y, Collington J. Computed tomography of metastatic lymph nodes. Arch Otolaryngol Head Neck Surg. ; 116:1190–1193

[159] Myers EN, Fagan JF. Management of the neck in cancer of the larynx. Ann Otol Rhinol Laryngol. ; 108(9):828–832

[160] Myers EN, Fagan JJ. Treatment of the N+neck in squamous cell carcinoma of the upper aerodigestive tract. Otolaryngol Clin North Am. ; 31(4):671–686

[161] Myers LL, Wax MK. Positron emission tomography in the evaluation of the negative neck in patients with oral cavity cancer. J Otolaryngol. ; 27(6):342–347

[162] Nahum AM, Mullally W, Marmor L. A syndrome resulting from radical neck dissection. Arch Otolaryngol. ; 74:424–428

[163] Narayan K, Crane CH, Kleid S, Hughes PG, Peters LJ. Planned neck dissection as an adjunct to the management of patients with advanced neck disease treated with definitive radiotherapy: for some or for all? Head Neck. ; 21(7):606–613

[164] Nowaczyk MT. [Lymphorrhea after neck dissection]. Otolaryngol Pol. ; 53(3):271–273

[165] O'Brien CJ, Smith JW, Soong SJ, Urist MM, Maddox WA. Neck dissection with and without radiotherapy: prognostic factors, patterns of recurrence, and survival. Am J Surg. ; 152(4):456–463

[166] O'Brien CJ, Urist MM, Maddox WA. Modified radical neck dissection. Terminology, technique, and indications. Am J Surg. ; 153(3):310–316

[167] Ogura JH, Biller HF, Wette R. Elective neck dissection for pharyngeal and laryngeal cancers. An evaluation. Ann Otol Rhinol Laryngol. ; 80(5):646–650

[168] Ohtawa T, Katagiri M, Harada T. A study of sternocleidomastoid muscular atrophy after modified neck dissection. Surg Today. ; 28(1):46–58

[169] Olofsson J, Tytor M. Complications in neck dissection. ORL J Otorhinolaryngol Relat Spec. ; 47(3):123–130

[170] Olsen KD, Caruso M, Foote RL, et al. Primary head and neck cancer. Histopathologic predictors of recurrence after neck dissection in patients with lymph node involvement. Arch Otolaryngol Head Neck Surg. ; 120(12):1370–1374

[171] Olsen KD. Reexamining the treatment of advanced laryngeal cancer. Head Neck. ; 32(1):1–7

[172] Pazos GA, Leonard DW, Blice J, Thompson DH. Blindness after bilateral neck dissection: case report and review. Am J Otolaryngol. ; 20(5):340–345

[173] Pearlman NW, Meyers AD, Sullivan WG. Modified radical neck dissection for squamous carcinoma of the head and neck. Surg Gynecol Obstet. ; 154(2):214–216

[174] Pellitteri PK, Robbins KT, Neuman T. Expanded application of selective neck dissection with regard to nodal status. Head Neck. ; 19(4):260–265

[175] Pendjer I, Mikić A, Golubić I, Vucicević S. Neck dissection in the management of regional metastases in patients with undifferentiated nasopharyngeal carcinomas. Eur Arch Otorhinolaryngol. ; 256(7):356–360

[176] Pernkopf FE. Topografische Anatomie des Menschen, Vol 3. Wien, Austria: Urban & Schwarzenburg; 1952

[177] Persky MS, Lagmay VM. Treatment of the clinically negative neck in oral squamous cell carcinoma. Laryngoscope. ; 109(7, Pt 1):1160–1164

[178] Peters LJ. The efficacy of postoperative radiotherapy for advanced head and neck cancer: quality of the evidence. Int J Radiat Oncol Biol Phys. ; 40(3):527–528

[179] Piccirillo JF. Importance of comorbidity in head and neck cancer. Laryngoscope. ; 110(4):593–602

[180] Pignon JP, Bourhis J, Domenge C, Designé L. Chemotherapy added to locoregional treatment for head and neck squamous-cell carcinoma: three meta-analyses of updated individual data. MACH-NC Collaborative Group. Meta-analysis of chemotherapy on head and neck cancer. Lancet. ; 355(9208):949–955

[181] Pignon JP, le Maître A, Maillard E, Bourhis J, MACH-NC Collaborative Group. Meta-analysis of chemotherapy in head and neck cancer (MACH-NC): an update on 93 randomised trials and 17,346 patients. Radiother Oncol. ; 92(1):4–14

[182] Pillsbury HC, III, Clark M. A rationale for therapy of the N0 neck. Laryngoscope. ; 107(10):1294–1315

[183] Pitman KT, Johnson JT, Myers EN. Effectiveness of selective neck dissection for management of the clinically negative neck. Arch Otolaryngol Head Neck Surg. ; 123(9):917–922

[184] Pointreau Y, Garaud P, Chapet S, et al. Randomized trial of induction chemotherapy with cisplatin and 5-fluorouracil with or without docetaxel for larynx preservation. J Natl Cancer Inst. ; 101(7):498–506

[185] Prim MP, de Diego JI, Fernández-Zubillaga A, García-Raya P, Madero R, Gavilán J. Patency and flow of the internal jugular vein after functional neck dissection. Laryngoscope. ; 110(1):47–50

[186] Prim MP, De Diego JI, Hardisson D, Madero R, Nistal M, Gavilán J. Extracapsular spread and desmoplastic pattern in neck lymph nodes: two prognostic factors of laryngeal cancer. Ann Otol Rhinol Laryngol. ; 108(7, Pt 1):672–676

[187] Redaelli de Zinis LO, Piccioni LO, Ghizzardi D, Mantini G, Antonelli AR. [Indications for elective neck dissection in malignant epithelial parotid tumors]. Acta Otorhinolaryngol Ital. ; 18(1):11–15

[188] Remmler D, Byers R, Scheetz J, et al. A prospective study of shoulder disability resulting from radical and modified neck dissections. Head Neck Surg. ; 8(4):280–286

[189] Righi M, Manfredi R, Farneti G, Pasquini E, Cenacchi V. Short-term versus long-term antimicrobial prophylaxis in oncologic head and neck surgery. Head Neck. ; 18(5):399–404

[190] Righi PD, Kopecky KK, Caldemeyer KS, Ball VA, Weisberger EC, Radpour S. Comparison of ultrasound-fine needle aspiration and computed tomography in patients undergoing elective neck dissection. Head Neck. ; 19(7):604–610

[191] Robbins KT, Clayman G, Levine PA, et al. American Head and Neck Society, American Academy of Otolaryngology–Head and Neck Surgery. Neck dissection classification update: revisions proposed by the American Head and Neck Society and the American Academy of Otolaryngology-Head and Neck Surgery. Arch Otolaryngol Head Neck Surg. ; 128(7):751–758

[192] Robbins KT, Favrot S, Hanna D, Cole R. Risk of wound infection in patients with head and neck cancer. Head Neck. ; 12(2):143–148

[193] Robbins KT, Medina JE, Wolfe GT, Levine PA, Sessions RB, Pruet CW. Standardizing neck dissection terminology: official report of the Academy's Committee for Head and Neck Surgery and Oncology. Arch Otolaryngol Head Neck Surg. ; 117(6):601–605

[194] Robbins KT, Shaha AR, Medina JE, et al. Committee for Neck Dissection Classification, American Head and Neck Society. Consensus statement on the classification and terminology of neck dissection. Arch Otolaryngol Head Neck Surg. ; 134(5):536–538

[195] Robbins KT. Classification of neck dissection: current concepts and future considerations. Otolaryngol Clin North Am. ; 31(4):639–655

[196] Rodrigo JP, Alvarez JC, Gómez JR, Suárez C, Fernández JA, Martínez JA. Comparison of three prophylactic antibiotic regimens in clean-contaminated head and neck surgery. Head Neck. ; 19(3):188–193

[197] Roy PH, Beahrs OH. Spinal accessory nerve in radical neck dissections. Am J Surg. ; 118(5):800–804

[198] Saffold SH, Wax MK, Nguyen A, et al. Sensory changes associated with selective neck dissection. Arch Otolaryngol Head Neck Surg. ; 126(3):425–428

[199] Saunders JR, Jr, Hirata RM, Jaques DA. Considering the spinal accessory nerve in head and neck surgery. Am J Surg. ; 150(4):491–494

[200] Schuller DE, Platz CE, Krause CJ. Spinal accessory lymph nodes: a prospective study of metastatic involvement. Laryngoscope. ; 88(3):439–450

[201] Schuller DE, Reiches NA, Hamaker RC, et al. Analysis of disability resulting from treatment including radical neck dissection or modified neck dissection. Head Neck Surg. ; 6(1):551–558

[202] Schultes G, Gaggl A, Kärcher H. Reconstruction of accessory nerve defects with vascularized long thoracic vs. non-vascularized thoracodorsal nerve. J Reconstr Microsurg. ; 15(4):265–270, discussion 270–271

[203] Shah JP, Andersen PE. The impact of patterns of nodal metastasis on modifications of neck dissection. Ann Surg Oncol. ; 1(6):521–532

[204] Shah JP, Medina JE, Shaha AR, Schantz SP, Marti JR. Cervical lymph node metastasis. Curr Probl Surg. ; 30(3):1–335

[205] Shah JP, Strong E, Spiro RH, Vikram B. Surgical grand rounds. Neck dissection: current status and future possibilities. Clin Bull. ; 11(1):25–33

[206] Shah JP. Cervical lymph node metastases–diagnostic, therapeutic, and prognostic implications. Oncology (Williston Park). ; 4(10):61–69, discussion 72, 76

[207] Shah JP. Patterns of cervical lymph node metastasis from squamous carcinomas of the upper aerodigestive tract. Am J Surg. ; 160(4):405–409

[208] Shaha AR. Management of the neck in thyroid cancer. Otolaryngol Clin North Am. ; 31(5):823–831

[209] Sheppard IJ, Watkinson JC, Glaholm J. Conservation surgery in head and neck cancer. Clin Otolaryngol Allied Sci. ; 23(5):385–387

[210] Shingaki S, Nomura T, Takada M, Kobayashi T, Suzuki I, Nakajima T. The impact of extranodal spread of lymph node metastases in patients with oral cancer. Int J Oral Maxillofac Surg. ; 28(4):279–284

[211] Short SO, Kaplan JN, Laramore GE, Cummings CW. Shoulder pain and function after neck dissection with or without preservation of the spinal accessory nerve. Am J Surg. ; 148(4):478–482

7

[212] Silvestre-Benis C. Consideraciones sobre el problema del tratamiento quirúrgico de los ganglios en los cánceres de la laringe. Actas II Congreso Sudamericano ORL. Montevideo, Uruguay; 1944

[213] Sist T, Miner M, Lema M. Characteristics of postradical neck pain syndrome: a report of 25 cases. J Pain Symptom Manage. ; 18(2):95–102

[214] Skolnik EM, Deutsch EC. Conservative neck dissection. J Laryngol Otol Suppl. ; 8 Suppl:105

[215] Skolnik EM, Katz AH, Becker SP, Mantravadi R, Stal S. Evolution of the clinically negative neck. Ann Otol Rhinol Laryngol. ; 89(6, Pt 1):551–555

[216] Skolnik EM, Tenta LT, Wineinger DM, Tardy ME, Jr. Preservation of XI cranial nerve in neck dissections. Laryngoscope. ; 77(8):1304–1314

[217] Smullen JL, Lejeune FE, Jr. Complications of neck dissection. J La State Med Soc. ; 151(11):544–547

[218] Snow GB, Patel P, Leemans CR, Tiwari R. Management of cervical lymph nodes in patients with head and neck cancer. Eur Arch Otorhinolaryngol. ; 249(4):187–194

[219] Sobol S, Jensen C, Sawyer W, II, Costiloe P, Thong N. Objective comparison of physical dysfunction after neck dissection. Am J Surg. ; 150(4):503–509

[220] Som PM, Curtin HD, Mancuso AA. An imaging-based classification for the cervical nodes designed as an adjunct to recent clinically based nodal classifications. Arch Otolaryngol Head Neck Surg. ; 125(4):388–396

[221] Som PM. The present controversy over the imaging method of choice for evaluating the soft tissues of the neck. AJNR Am J Neuroradiol. ; 18(10):1869–1872

[222] Soo KC, Guiloff RJ, Oh A, Della Rovere GQ, Westbury G. Innervation of the trapezius muscle: a study in patients undergoing neck dissections. Head Neck. ; 12(6):488–495

[223] Spiro JD, Spiro RH, Strong EW. The management of chyle fistula. Laryngoscope. ; 100(7):771–774

[224] Spiro RH, Strong EW, Shah JP. Classification of neck dissection: variations on a new theme. Am J Surg. ; 168(5):415–418

[225] Stack BC, Jr, Ferris RL, Goldenberg D, et al. American Thyroid Association Surgical Affairs Committee. American Thyroid Association consensus review and statement regarding the anatomy, terminology, and rationale for lateral neck dissection in differentiated thyroid cancer. Thyroid. ; 22(5):501–508

[226] Steinkamp HJ, van der Hoeck E, Böck JC, Felix R. [The extracapsular spread of cervical lymph node metastases: the diagnostic value of computed tomography]. RoFo Fortschr Geb Rontgenstr Nuklearmed. ; 170(5):457–462

[227] Stell PM. Adjuvant chemotherapy in head and neck cancer. Semin Radiat Oncol. ; 2(3):195–205

[228] Stell PM. The management of cervical lymph nodes in head and neck cancer. Proc R Soc Med. ; 68(2):83–85

[229] Stenson KM, Haraf DJ, Pelzer H, et al. The role of cervical lymphadenectomy after aggressive concomitant chemoradiotherapy: the feasibility of selective neck dissection. Arch Otolaryngol Head Neck Surg. ; 126(8):950–956

[230] Strong MS, Vaughan CW, Kayne HL, et al. A randomized trial of preoperative radiotherapy in cancer of the oropharynx and hypopharynx. Am J Surg. ; 136(4):494–500

[231] Suárez C, Llorente JL, Nuñez F, Díaz C, Gomez J. Neck dissection with or without postoperative radiotherapy in supraglottic carcinomas. Otolaryngol Head Neck Surg. ; 109(1):3–9

[232] Suárez O. El problema de las metastasis linfáticas y alejadas del cancer de laringe e hipofaringe. Rev Otorrinolaringol. ; 23:83–99

[233] Talmi YP, Horowitz Z, Pfeffer MR, et al. Pain in the neck after neck dissection. Otolaryngol Head Neck Surg. ; 123(3):302–306

[234] Talmi YP. Minimizing complications in neck dissection. J Laryngol Otol. ; 113 (2):101–113

[235] Terrell JE, Fisher SG, Wolf GT, The Veterans Affairs Laryngeal Cancer Study Group. Long-term quality of life after treatment of laryngeal cancer. Arch Otolaryngol Head Neck Surg. ; 124(9):964–971

[236] Terrell JE, Welsh DE, Bradford CR, et al. Pain, quality of life, and spinal accessory nerve status after neck dissection. Laryngoscope. ; 110(4):620–626

[237] Terz JJ, Lawrence W Jr. Ineffectiveness of combined therapy (radiation and surgery) in the management of malignancies of the oral cavity, larynx, and pharynx. In: Kagan AR, Miles JW, eds. Head and Neck Oncology: Controversies in Cancer Treatment. Boston, MA: GK Hall Medical Publishers; 1981:110–125

[238] Thomas GR, Greenberg J, Wu KT, et al. Planned early neck dissection before radiation for persistent neck nodes after induction chemotherapy. Laryngoscope. ; 107(8):1129–1137

[239] Timon CV, Brown D, Gullane P. Internal jugular vein blowout complicating head and neck surgery. J Laryngol Otol. ; 108(5):423–425

[240] Traynor SJ, Cohen JI, Gray J, Andersen PE, Everts EC. Selective neck dissection and the management of the node-positive neck. Am J Surg. ; 172(6):654–657

[241] Truffert P. Le cou: Anatomie Topographique: Les Aponévroses, Les Loges. Paris: Librairie Arnette; 1922

[242] Tschammler A, Ott G, Schang T, Seelbach-Goebel B, Schwager K, Hahn D. Lymphadenopathy: differentiation of benign from malignant disease–color Doppler US assessment of intranodal angioarchitecture. Radiology. ; 208(1):117–123

[243] Tu GY. Upper neck (level II) dissection for N0 neck supraglottic carcinoma. Laryngoscope. ; 109(3):467–470

[244] Umeda M, Nishimatsu N, Teranobu O, Shimada K. Criteria for diagnosing lymph node metastasis from squamous cell carcinoma of the oral cavity: a study of the relationship between computed tomographic and histologic findings and outcome. J Oral Maxillofac Surg. ; 56(5):585–593, discussion 593–595

[245] Valdés Olmos RA, Koops W, Loftus BM, et al. Correlative 201Tl SPECT, MRI and ex vivo 201Tl uptake in detecting and characterizing cervical lymphadenopathy in head and neck squamous cell carcinoma. J Nucl Med. ; 40(9):1414–1419

[246] Vallejo Valdezate L, Díaz Suárez I, De Las Heras P, Cuetos M, Gil-Carcedo García LM. Consideraciones anatómicas sobre la importancia de la rama externa del nervio espinal en la cirugía del triángulo posterior del cuello. Acta Otorrinolaringol Esp. ; 50(8):630–634

[247] van Leeuwen PA, Sauerwein HP, Kuik DJ, Snow GB, Quak JJ. Assessment of malnutrition parameters in head and neck cancer and their relation to postoperative complications. Head Neck. ; 19:419–425

[248] van den Brekel MW, Castelijns JA, Reitsma LC, Leemans CR, van der Waal I, Snow GB. Outcome of observing the N0 neck using ultrasonographic-guided cytology for follow-up. Arch Otolaryngol Head Neck Surg. ; 125(2):153–156

[249] van den Brekel MW, van der Waal I, Meijer CJ, Freeman JL, Castelijns JA, Snow GB. The incidence of micrometastases in neck dissection specimens obtained from elective neck dissections. Laryngoscope. ; 106(8):987–991

[250] Vandenbrouck C, Sancho-Garnier H, Chassagne D, Saravane D, Cachin Y, Micheau C. Elective versus therapeutic radical neck dissection in epidermoid carcinoma of the oral cavity: results of a randomized clinical trial. Cancer. ; 46(2):386–390

[251] Vikram B, Strong EW, Shah JP, Spiro R. Failure in the neck following multimodality treatment for advanced head and neck cancer. Head Neck Surg. ; 6(3):724–729

[252] Vikram B. Selective neck dissection. Arch Otolaryngol Head Neck Surg. ; 124 (9):1044–1045

[253] Vokes EE, Weichselbaum RR, Lippman SM, Hong WK. Head and neck cancer. N Engl J Med. ; 328(3):184–194

[254] Vokes EE. Combined-modality therapy of head and neck cancer. Oncology (Williston Park). ; 11(9) Suppl 9:27–30

[255] Ward GE, Robben JO. A composite operation for radical neck dissection and removal of cancer of the mouth. Cancer. ; 4(1):98–109

[256] Weber PC, Johnson JT, Myers EN. Impact of bilateral neck dissection on recovery following supraglottic laryngectomy. Arch Otolaryngol Head Neck Surg. ; 119(1):61–64

[257] Weber RS, Berkey BA, Forastiere A, et al. Outcome of salvage total laryngectomy following organ preservation therapy: the Radiation Therapy Oncology Group trial 91–11. Arch Otolaryngol Head Neck Surg. ; 129(1):44–49

[258] Weber RS, Hankins P, Rosenbaum B, Raad I. Nonwound infections following head and neck oncologic surgery. Laryngoscope. ; 103(1, Pt 1):22–27

[259] Weisman RA, Robbins KT. Management of the neck in patients with head and neck cancer treated by concurrent chemotherapy and radiation. Otolaryngol Clin North Am. ; 31(5):773–784

[260] Weitz JW, Weitz SL, McElhinney AJ. A technique for preservation of spinal accessory nerve function in radical neck dissection. Head Neck Surg. ; 5(1):75–78

[261] Werner JA. Aktueller Stand der Versorgung des Lymphabflusses maligner Kopf-Hals-Tumoren. In: Deutsche Gesellschaft fur Hals-Nasen-Ohrenheilkunde, Kopf- und Hals-Chirurgie. Springer-Verlag; 1997

[262] Weymuller EA, Jr. Rationale for elective modified neck dissection: a word of caution. Head Neck. ; 11(1):93–94

[263] Wide JM, White DW, Woolgar JA, Brown JS, Vaughan ED, Lewis-Jones HG. Magnetic resonance imaging in the assessment of cervical nodal metastasis in oral squamous cell carcinoma. Clin Radiol. ; 54(2):90–94

[264] Withers HR, Peters LJ, Taylor JM. Dose-response relationship for radiation therapy of subclinical disease. Int J Radiat Oncol Biol Phys. ; 31(2):353–359

7

Suggested Readings

[265] Wolf GT, Fisher SG. Effectiveness of salvage neck dissection for advanced regional metastases when induction chemotherapy and radiation are used for organ preservation. Laryngoscope. ; 102(8):934–939

[266] Woods JE, Yugueros P. A safe and rapid technique for modified neck dissection. Ann Plast Surg. ; 43(1):90–95

[267] Wustrow TP. [Personal experiences. On the nomenclature of various forms of neck dissection]. Laryngorhinootologie. ; 68(9):529–530

[268] Yang CY, Andersen PE, Everts EC, Cohen JI. Nodal disease in purely glottic carcinoma: is elective neck treatment worthwhile? Laryngoscope. ; 108(7): 1006–1008

[269] Yii NW, Patel SG, Rhys-Evans PH, Breach NM. Management of the N0 neck in early cancer of the oral tongue. Clin Otolaryngol Allied Sci. ; 24(1):75–79

[270] Yii NW, Patel SG, Williamson P, Breach NM. Use of apron flap incision for neck dissection. Plast Reconstr Surg. ; 103(6):1655–1660

[271] Yuen AP, Lam KY, Chan AC, et al. Clinicopathological analysis of elective neck dissection for N0 neck of early oral tongue carcinoma. Am J Surg. ; 177(1): 90–92

[272] Yuen AP, Wei WI, Wong YM, Tang KC. Elective neck dissection versus observation in the treatment of early oral tongue carcinoma. Head Neck. ; 19 (7):583–588

[273] Zupi A, Califano L, Mangone GM, Longo F, Piombino P. Surgical management of the neck in squamous cell carcinoma of the floor of the mouth. Oral Oncol. ; 34(6):472–475

7

Index

Note: Page numbers set **bold** or *italic* indicate headings or figures, respectively.

Index